THE PUZZLE OF
PAIN

THE PUZZLE OF

PAIN

Translated from the French edition
by Fideline A. Djité-Bruce

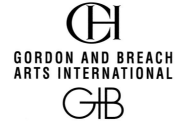

GORDON AND BREACH
ARTS INTERNATIONAL

First published in 1992 in the French language by
Gordon and Breach Science Publishers S.A.,Y-Parc,
Chemin de la Sallaz, 1400 Yverdon, Suisse

First published in the English language in 1994 by
G+B Arts International Limited
Distributed in Australia by Craftsman House
20 Barcoo Street
East Roseville, NSW 2069, Australia

Distributed internationally through the following offices:

EUROPE
G+B Arts International (Europe) Ltd
St Johanns-Vorstadt 19
Postfach 4004 Basel Switzerland

USA
STBS LTD.
PO Box 786
Cooper Station New York NY 10276

ASIA
STBS (Singapore) Pte Ltd
25 Tannery Road
Singapore 1334
Republic of Singapore

ISBN 976 8097 89 2

Design Stephen Smedley
Printer Kyodo, Singapore

Contents

Hello, I am PAIN

I'M amazed you want to read about me. Normally you try to avoid me and when I do arrive, you desperately want me to fade into the background or completely disappear, and sometimes even imagine you can forget me …

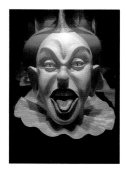

But ever since the beginning, I've dogged man's every step. Throughout his existence, I've circled unrelentingly, waiting for my chance to leap out of the darkness and seize him by the throat. I am present from the first breath of the newborn baby. I reappear with every disorder and disease, surging out of every wound, and I return at the last breath, to break into my victim's dying thoughts and to torture his soul.

I'm also there in your loves and friendships, lurking behind every emotion. When your loved one leaves for an hour, a year or forever, it's me, PAIN, that grips your heart and leaves you breathless and trembling. I'm the one who makes you wring your hands and brings tears to your eyes.

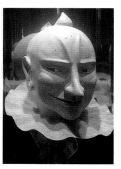

I live in memory, embellishing myths and legends. My presence spans religions and philosophies. I loom up to darken the future and banish hope, eroding your will to go on. And I barge into the present moment of each and every one of you, to splinter your existence and thwart your ambitions.

No one escapes, because I am PAIN. I make the child cry and the adult curse. I assail men and women, indifferently. The rich can buy no indulgence, the poor are condemned to endure my torment. I am everywhere: in the worker's tools, in the sculptor's hands, in the painter's eyes, in the melody of the musician, on the blank sheet before the writer's poised pen. I erupt on your movie and television screens. At night, I trouble your dreams.

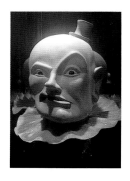

Why, then, do you want to know more about me?

Is it to solve the riddle of who I am? Is it to learn my weaknesses? To know how to avoid me? How to dominate me? To tame me?

Very well, then, read on. But remember that I will be your constant companion. Welcome to my dominion! I am PAIN.

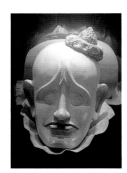

Extract from the text spoken by the puppet symbolising pain which animated the exhibition
La Douleur *organised by the Institut pour la Cooperation Scientifique Internationale presented at the Cité des Sciences et l'Industrie de la Villette, Paris.*

Sculptures by Jean-Lionel Breuil
Photography by Michel Lamoureux

Authors

Robert T. Anderson — *Professor of Anthropology, Mills College, Oakland, California*

Scott T. Anderson — *Assistant Professor of Medicine, Uniformed Services, University of the Health Services, Bethesda, Maryland*

Allan I. Basbaum — *Professor of Anatomy and Physiology, University of California, San Francisco*

Jean-Marie Besson — *Director of the Physiological and Pharmacological Research Laboratories on the Nervous System, INSERM, Paris*

Francois Boureau — *Director of the Centre for the Evaluation and the Treatment of Pain, Saint-Antoine Hospital, Paris*

Georges Duby — *Professor at the College de France, Paris*

Michel Enaudeau — *Journalist, Paris*

Jan Gybels — *Professor of Neurology and Neurosurgery, University of Louvain*

Patrick Lacoste — *Psychoanalyst, Bordeaux, Lecturer at the University of Paris VII*

Marc Le Bot — *Professor at the University Panthéon-Sorbonne, Paris*

Jean-Paul Natali — *Neurobiologist, Research Fellow in the Sciences and Techniques of Museums, Cité des Sciences et de l'Industrie, La Villette, Paris*

Roy Porter — *Senior Research Fellow, Wellcome Institute for the History of Medicine, London*

Bernard P. Roques — *Director of the Department of Molecular Chemistry and Pharmacy, University René Descartes, Paris*

Jean-Didier Vincent — *Director of the Alfred Fessard Institute, CNRS, Paris*

ix

Foreword

Geneviève and Maurice Lévy

THIS book was prompted by an exhibition on Pain, organised by the Institute for International Scientific Co-operation in Paris in 1992-1993. Some of the contributions in this volume draw their inspiration directly from the themes of the exhibition and were written by distinguished specialists who are members of the Scientific Council. The remainder of the book explores other aspects of the human experience of pain, such as artistic creativity, history, anthropology, philosophy, psychoanalysis and literature.

Pain as a focus of interest may seem a novelty. Yet it has been the theme of many research projects, of seminars, congresses and books. In 1973, the International Association for the Study of Pain was established.

The 'male dominated middle ages' despised and suppressed the suffering of the body. The Western world, for a long time, also imposed a convenient silence on the subject of pain. As for medical science, it has always been interested in the pathologies and the symptoms rather than in pain *per se*. Today this new interest in the subject of pain is much more than the result of media promotion. Rather it is the beginning of a revolution in medical thought and in the approach to pain by the patient and the relatives and friends.

Those changes are linked to the almost contagious spread of what the present-day Western world calls 'chronic intractable pain': pain that resists any type of treatment, which leaves one simply at a loss, and diagnosis of which essentially relies on the patient's description and complaint.

Pain is expensive, in every sense of the word, for society and for the individual whose life is transformed into a nightmare. One is subjected to the atrocious and expects the worst with a feeling of powerlessness and with no hope of a way out. And since one cannot incessantly complain, one ends up retreating into absolute silence and the psychological balance is also affected. Even though it is not fatal, in this sense chronic pain is very dangerous.

The International Association for the Study of Pain defines pain as follows:

'A sensorial and *emotional* experience associated with a real or potential tissue damage or *described* in such terms.'

In this now universally accepted definition of pain, the words in italics are important. Thus, the main thing is that the pain is physically experienced by the individual concerned. The patient is taken at his or her word. Pain is not just in the head.

Hence, pain is no longer just the sign (to be respected) of a pathological reality (yet to be discovered). It becomes a diagnosis, a medical category, and the therapeutics of it then take into account all of its various aspects: the physiological, the affective and the situational, including its largely incurable nature. What can be treated will be taken care of, helping the patient to live with what remains, probably for a long time.

The modern model of pain partially dissociated from its function as a sign, (which can degrade, dehumanise, destroy the person), helps to free pain's 'good' aspects. Anything that can be attributed to pain in terms of value – for instance courage, sacrifice, better self knowledge, creativity, spiritual elevation – can no longer disguise its absolute harmfulness. Even the traditional association between women and suffering is challenged. Women now accept, with decreasing guilt, not giving birth in pain. The pain of giving birth is no longer perceived as a form of 'beautiful pain'. Even if the myth of good suffering has left its marks, Job, the symbol of the biblical resignation to suffering, has become the enemy; one has to rebel, to defend oneself against pain. It is no longer acceptable to be told: 'that's life'. Preaching the acceptance of pain to others is seen as a form of oppression. All pain that can be avoided must be avoided. In our hedonistic cultures, the change from law to norm is a very fast one: the duty is no longer to accept pain, but rather to refuse it and run away from it.

One tends to drift, insidiously, from destructive pain, which science must relieve, to the structuring pain that is integral to life. Too much physical pain is destructive and too much psychical pain can hinder the thought process. Does that mean that we are to forget that we must live with some pain? Does it mean that we should forget that there is an unavoidable pain for the mind of the child to be alerted to reality and early learning? Or that the congenital inability to feel pain is absolutely inhuman and that pain remains the basis of diagnosis and a necessary alarm for the living?

There is a threshold below which pain must be tolerated but beyond which it becomes an act of violence and overwhelms the individual. This threshold varies according to each individual. It is up to the patient and especially to the practitioner to assess this limit in a context where there is no clear cut boundary between the body and the spirit. Pain is becoming a medical speciality in its own right. That will no doubt increasingly continue to be the case.

Pain: Beyond all Paradoxes

Jean-Paul Natali

'Happiness is only a dream whereas pain is real.'

Voltaire, *Candide*

WHAT is pain?

What is its purpose? How can we get rid of it? Why must I suffer?

These are some of the questions that concern each and every one of us and that have been asked since the dawn of time. In trying to answer these questions, one immediately realises that, beyond the evidence of our own pain, the ancestral anxiety concerning this unknown comes forward again. And we can only catch a glimpse of it. We still fail to understand the human essence, and our ignorance of pain is part of this failure.

How then can we tackle the study of pain? It might seem as though I know what I feel when I am in pain, but I have yet to gain a real understanding of the feelings others experience when they are in pain. In other words, are we capable of studying pain in objective terms so as to grasp its general nature? Pain, in this context, is part of the enigma of our consciousness. Any attempt to make a judgement about it tends to drive it back into an 'abyss' and leads us into some strange paradoxes.

Firstly, as has already been stated, pain is both fundamentally universal and strictly individual. It is universal because no one can escape it, and individual because each of us has our own experience of it. And this experience is different from any other. In this sense, it appears to be complementary with death, which it often accompanies. Thus, in spite of our will to escape it, it remains an integral part of our status as human beings. It is a component of us and only takes on meaning through us.

We also know that pain can be shared but not exchanged. Other people can only cause me, by empathy, to feel pain in seeing them suffer; but it is impossible for them to pass on to me this suffering exactly as they feel it. We cannot really communicate at this level. All I can do is guess, through recollections of my own suffering, what the other person is desperately trying to express through their behaviour, gestures and words. The pain of others and what I may come to know about it are only within the realm of my own subjectivity. While we cannot ignore the existence of pain with regard to the person who is suffering, paradoxically, we cannot feel it in its reality. We know nothing of this pain and can only recall a personal enactment of it. Thus pain appears as one of the measures of this double limit: firstly, our need to communicate and, secondly, our inability to satisfy this need.

Thus there exists the need to implement a truly scientific approach in order to try to understand and define pain, its causes and its origins. We may have to settle for the following definition proposed by the International Association for the Study of Pain (IASP): 'Pain is an unpleasant sensorial and emotional experience associated with a real or potential tissue damage or described in such terms.'[1]

Defining pain as a sensation and an emotion implies a separation of the biological mechanism (nociception) from its awareness (pain). For the researcher who takes interest in the structure of its intimate mechanisms, the evidence of painful perception disappears in the face of the complexity of the biological being. When this being is reduced to cellular dynamics and molecular exchanges, pain loses its primary meaning to become a profusion of nervous signals dependent upon the release of neuro-hormones. It is not clear what this will lead to with regard to the affect and rationality of the person who is suffering. Paradoxically, at this point, the object of study gives way to the study of the object.

In other words, in order to be coherent, biological science is forced to study only the objective aspect of the phenomenon and to ignore the subjectivity of the state of consciousness which results from it. But, as R. Melzack and P.D. Wall put it: 'A real understanding of the perception of pain goes beyond the problem of a lesion of tissue and the simple study of the sensorial signals of pain.'[2]

Therefore, this painful perception must be taken into account if one wishes to fight against it and eliminate it. And this is in fact the attitude that medical doctors must have. They first consider pain as the indicator of a dysfunction. It helps them make a diagnosis: the localisation, the nature and frequency of the manifestations of pain according to the patient often make it possible to formulate a first hypothesis, in the case of an illness in its early stages. The other actions, more or less empirical and more or less efficient, will follow from this and will try, beyond the pathological treatment, to soothe the suffering.

However, the medical doctor is sometimes confronted with a situation in which pain becomes the essential element of the illness. It takes hold to the point of becoming exclusively destructive. Paradoxically also, pain may reveal itself outside any known cause of illness and may remain intractable; in this case, it can challenge the available medical know-how as well as the pharmacological arsenal. Patients suffering from chronic pain see their bodies transformed into battle zones; they have no way of escaping the unbearable tyranny forced upon them by their pain. Medical doctors, nurses and assistant nurses

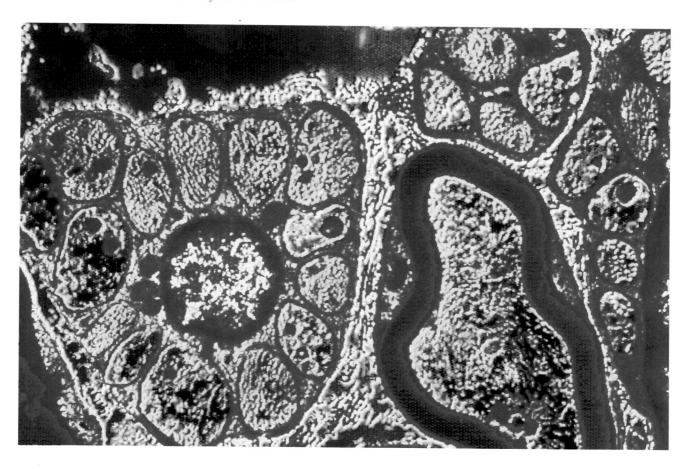

must therefore change their strategy and interact precisely with the mind of the patient. They must return to the humanity of the doctor/patient relationship that has sometimes been overwhelmed by technological progress and the demands of good performance and efficient management.

Finally, considering the personal development it provokes – including the evolution of human production which claims to be a result – pain seems absolutely necessary for the advancement of humanity. And this may be part of its paradox. One cannot ignore the fact that pain, beyond its immediate effects, plays an important role in human adaptation to the environment. Through the situations and difficulties pain constantly creates, it continually forces human beings to surpass themselves. Hence, physical pain creates anxieties which in turn, cause psychical pain; in so doing it modifies our perceptions of the world. In the process, the disinvestment of the self might result in a more objective and a better understanding of external reality. According to Freud: 'The change from physical to psychical pain is equivalent to the change from narcissistic investment to investment in the object.'[3]

Thus pain takes on an ontogenetic dimension that can be found in all civilisations. Hence for all children it is the foundation which builds them up or

Section of a neuron. Original computer graphics by Pierrick Van Thé. (Agence Liaisons)

destroys them. Its continuous presence hinders the development of the body and distorts the mind. And yet, fighting against it can shape character, foster endurance, teach about surpassing oneself, and can bring rewards. When pain is not present,[4] children's bodies are in danger in an environment where they have no understanding of their physical limits. In this particular instance, pain makes the world aggressive and incomprehensible to a child. And yet, escaping it is the necessary condition for a child to live a better life, to blossom and be fulfilled. As Boris Cyrulnik points out: '. . . the absence of pain is not structuring, neither is the excess of pain; and. . . pain is necessary for the structuring; that is the case for man. . . for the animal, so long as it is charged with affect, and for man, so long as it is charged with affect and meaning.'[5]

We know very well that if we could completely rid ourselves of pain, we would, in the process, be eliminating an important part of our humanity. Nevertheless, it is quite normal to wish for a painless world.

As the reader might have concluded by now, our approach is neither a manichaean vision denouncing the calamities of pain nor a linear construction decrying its fatality. However, we do not want to give the impression that we accept either pain's tragedies or its inexorability. Beyond all the paradoxes pain creates, we must approach it from different perspectives, even if that means we end up breaking it down into special pieces and risk losing part of its reality.

The articles in this volume allow the reader to take stock of the current orientation of medical and scientific knowledge concerning pain. Nevertheless, we thought it necessary to point out some new ideas analysing pain in areas as diverse as history and the plastic arts. For pain is also an expression. For this reason, we have also decided to add to the words of the explanatory articles by including reproductions of pictorial works. This is not merely for the sake of having illustrations, but essentially to complement the rational response with the emotional.

To achieve this, we have followed the logic of the exhibition which inspired this book. Therefore readers should not expect this collection of papers to read like a didactic and encyclopedic treatise. Our objective here is different. The specialists who have contributed papers to this volume want to make readers aware of a number of current issues on the subject of pain and direct their attention to new findings in this area.

Pain as an Object of Scientific Knowledge

As we have seen, the study of pain in the field of biology leads the researcher to treat its underlying structures and dynamics in objective ways. But science cannot achieve its goal by merely trying to simplify its object of study. It is important for scientists always to keep in mind the overall dimension of the phenomenon that they are trying to understand; otherwise they run the risk of confusing a mechanistic model with the reality of their subject. This is very important for biologists. The living – a phenomenon which emerges from matter and from temporality – can only be understood as a continuous movement between the mechanisms and the whole picture of the phenomenon at hand. Therefore, before any description of the structures which generate the painful 'messages' can be provided, it is particularly important to point out that behind the object – pain – there is necessarily a subject who suffers.

Jean-Didier Vincent's paper successfully expresses the above, yet is by no means limited to this observation. He reminds us that pain is in fact an emotion and that as such it refers us to another manifestation, the manifestation of pleasure. Linking pain and pleasure, not only as a strict dialectical relationship, but as complementary to states of being that are part of our knowledge of the world, allows the biologist to return pain to the realm of reality. Only then can it regain its full meaning and play its role, particularly in the dynamic of opposing choices.

This said, we must enter the mechanistic world from where the sensation of pain emerges. Allan Basbaum describes the complexity of the phenomena which generate and modulate the nociceptive signal and which underlie the

Blue neuron and head. Original computer graphics by Pierrick Van Thé. (Agence Liaisons)

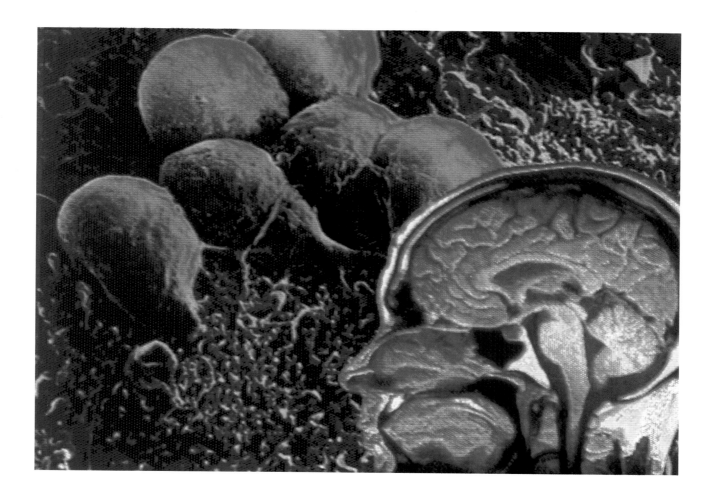

materiality of the message that the brain will end up integrating as a perception in its affective and rational configurations. Peripheral events, nerve impulses, chemical transmissions, ascending signals, competition between nerve fibres, descending modulations, affective mobilisations ... in short the neurophysiological history of pain, is part of an incredible complexity. Within the elements of this complexity one must search for and find the means, whether from physics and/or chemistry, that will be able to stop the painful 'message', so that it no longer reaches our consciousness.

Pain and Medical Practice

It is not surprising to find in the pharmacological approaches the difficulty of mastering the complex structures of this system. From which end should one tackle pain to reduce it? Should one be content with working on the periphery at the source of the stimulation, or should one operate on the transmission of the signal at the central level of the spinal cord and the brain? Should one make new molecules to be inserted in the various phases of the molecules at stake? Jean-Marie and Bernard Roques introduce us to their approach in the field of pharmacology. They tell us about the current directions of research and the expectations one can base on the future use of the progress made over the last few years.

But for the time being, pain is not so easy to brush aside. However, François Boureau tells us that a radical change has occurred in the practices within the clinics and in the area of medical ethics. Pain is fully acknowledged as a pathology in its own right. Anyone who expresses a feeling of pain is entitled to use all the available means to get rid of it.

All that remains is the identification of the different aspects and diverse causes of pain. And in this field of medicine, a new paradox emerges which may not be so new after all. The attention that the doctor gives the patient, the quality of the relationship with the patient, play an important role here. This role reminds us of the human and affective environments that medical technology has progressively abandoned. The emphasis is placed upon the importance of the 'psychological', not in order to send patients back to some kind of unscientific practice, but rather with a view to detecting the true affective components of their suffering. The doctor is forced to take notice of a 'placebo' relational effect which plays a major role in the patient's well being and 'recovery'. That is not all: for some years now a number of centres have been set up especially for the treatment of pain. When everything else failed, when it was acknowledged that, without co-operation, neither general practitioners nor specialists could reduce suffering on their own, pluridisciplinary teams began developing concerted strategies in which patients could actively participate and learn how to manage and negotiate their pain.

The fact remains that, in some cases, it is still necessary to resort to surgery. Jan Gybels tells us about the recent developments in this field. Destructive

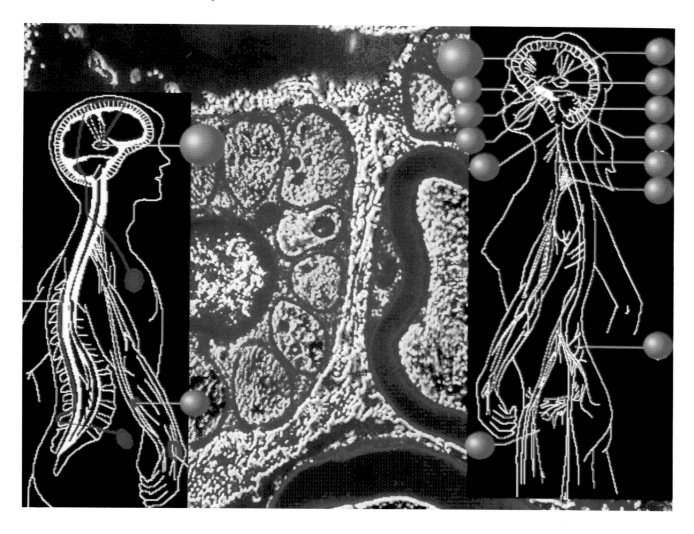

surgical operations are now a thing of the past. A new surgery of implantation allows for the steady administration of analgesic molecules such as morphines or the periodic stimulation of a number of central nervous centres. Along with the incredible development of medical imaging, surgery (though it remains exceptional in most cases) allows the patient to recover fully and enjoy the benefits of a normal social life in cases where other practices have failed.

Section of a man and a woman. Original computer graphics by Pierrick Van Thé. (Agence Liaisons)

Pain and its Social Context

Medicine today is actively engaged in the study of pain, but one must realise that, from a historical point of view, this is in fact a remarkable novelty. Georges Duby tries to give us a historical perspective of pain, pointing out the nature of some rare data he has been able to collect about the middle ages. It is not surprising to find that, once again, religion has had a major influence on the conception of physical pain. As divine punishment, and as a means of redemption, pain has been trivialised as an unavoidable human fact. It is still often not discussed and simply considered part of everyday life. And yet, pain is everywhere. It is expressed through the imitation of Jesus Christ, in the reproduction of the stigmata; it is particularly apparent in the representation of the Pietàs. The (human) pain is felt when one sees the suffering body of Christ, when one gazes upon the (divine) pain of the redeemer. This perception of pain inevitably conjures up other suffering bodies of a world contemporary with the Pietàs, a world undermined by wars, misery and epidemics.

And this is what one finds in the evolution of painting. Marc Le Bot reminds us that there is a tradition of the representation of pain through its different manifestations and in particular through the human cry which has often been used as a measure of painful states. These painful states are, in turn, associated with death. We have slowly moved from the state of 'Ecce Homo' to the distress of today's world. The representational expression of the past has given way to the distortion of faces and to the mutilation of bodies. In fact, art

Robot. Original computer graphics by Pierrick Van Thé.
(Agence Liaisons)

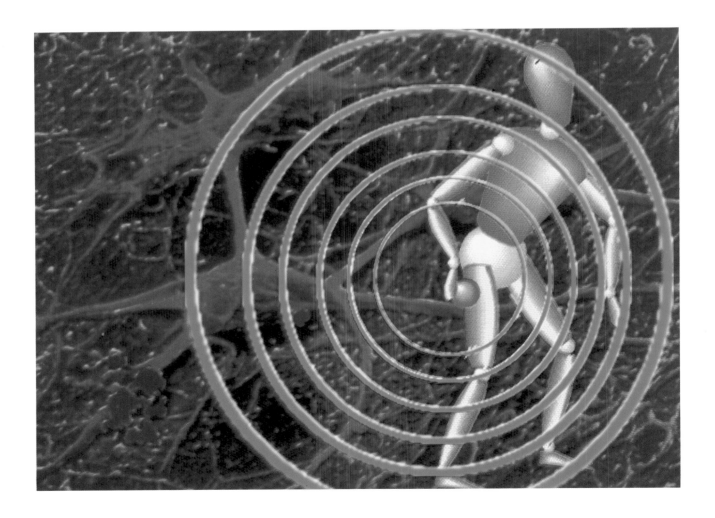

is a form of cultural expression intertwined with the reality of human societies. As such, it should now be a means for individuals to control their own destiny. Marc Le Bot leads us to see art as part of genuine social anthropology. Artists, witnesses of their time, would fully play a role in exploring and exhibiting the various pains our own evolution has in store for us.

Roy Porter points out the ambiguous relationships that Western societies have with pain. It is dreaded by the patient who experiences it. Western society also inflicts cruelty on outcasts, for the enlightenment of others, and in the education of children. Pain is a taboo subject, reflecting an elitist contempt for the flesh and its hardships. Paradoxically, it was during the Age of Enlightenment that the Anglo-Saxon world, shocked by the Cartesian theory regarding the insensitivity of animals, accentuated the protest against the suffering of others.

One of the great mysteries of pain is that it is a product of culture. The teachings of the ethnologists, reviewed by Robert and Scott Anderson with reference to contemporary social groups, remind us that there is very little variation in the neurology of pain with different genetic and racial characteristics. They also remind us that the considerable differences observed from one group of people to another in dealing with painful experiences, are connected with cultural attitudes. The historical and ethnographical literature is full of examples of 'euphoric' agonies, of atrocious suffering endured under hypnosis, of collective trances making possible all kinds of heroic acts. The authors claim that these rituals can produce biochemical responses which, by reducing the anxiety accompanying the pain, may reduce the sensation of the pain.

The Ontological Origin of Pain

It is claimed that acute pain can 'drive you mad'. But what is the nature of pain that does not express the usual logic of the body, pain that is intractable? According to Patrick Lacoste, apart from the psychological effect of the slightest physical pain, psychoanalysis distinguishes between psychogenetic pains of the body and psychical pains. Psychoanalysis also suggests that there are unconscious pains, in the same way that there are affects which can remain unconscious against all consciousness and rationalisation. In fact, the analytical clinic enables us to get closer to the psychical pain which is more innate than pain and suffering.

Sometimes this kind of demented pain can only be recalled by the diagram of the breakdown of the defences, because it actually concerns the permanent echo of a flaw in the makeup of the self. It is also about a void in the ability of being and thinking which cannot be reduced to a blank in the memory. This void can always reveal itself, provided it can be identified, and confront the analyst with innate pain, with the brutal perspective that the mind must go through in order simply to start.

Pain is therefore innate. Michel Enaudeau reminds us that, in philosophy,

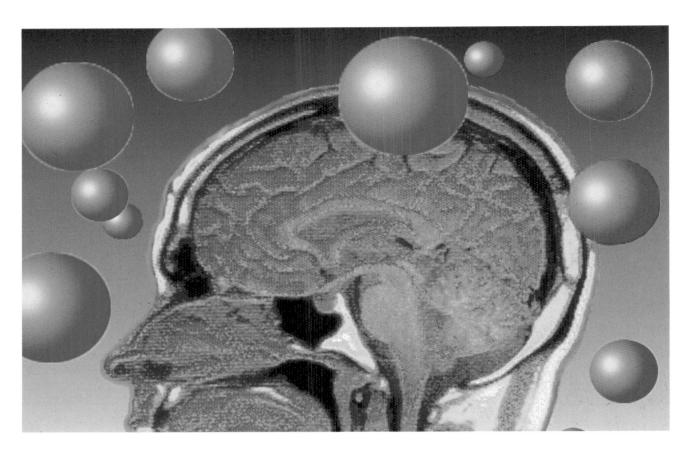

Head with bubbles. Original computer
graphics by Pierrick Van Thé.
(Agence Liaisons)

pleasure was perceived as the restoration of an order which was threatened by pain. This was the general and dominant line of thought from the Greeks through to Freud's first publications. As Descartes put it, one must have experienced pain in order to feel pleasure, just as one must have a concept of the infinite in order to be able to imagine finitude.

Is there, for the wise person, a positive use of pain that would differ from Pascal's definition, that could be endured as a prerequisite to happiness as Epicurus sees it, or be an incentive for action as Kant would have it? Can it be understood within the self, as introduction, or conversion into another order, without being imposed to the other through education?

Pain as a Special State of Mind

It could be literature that has provided a better analysis of pain. The writer, who is master of both personal intimacy and world consciousness, projects visions of a personal experience of pain that are sometimes accurate and often touching. The written word has the ability to evoke the underlying emotion that is felt when one is confronted with pain. Striking examples of the description of the effects of painful states can be found in literature of all genres and forms. It should be pointed out here that J.M.G. Le Clézio's wonderful book[6] strongly influenced the idea for the exhibition that the present volume is based on. The description of the evolution of the character who is suffering (Beaumont) provides a good example of the changes in the states of consciousness that come with the onset of painful situations.

Finally it must be stressed that discussing pain is one of the rare means through which the individual's ability suddenly to cope with a 'different state of being' can be shown. To suffer often means that one has to alter completely one's relationship with the world. One lives differently, understands things in a different way and expresses a 'familiarly strange' personality with which one can identify without really being able to understand. One becomes confused and this adds to the anguish of suffering.

However, experiencing pain is still annoying and one would like to avoid it. Nevertheless, when in pain it is sometimes possible to reconsider, through the distorted filter that it provides, the reassuring positions we have progressively negotiated with life. Maybe it is cruel to realise that 'happiness is only a dream whereas pain is real'.

Pain gives us a lopsided vision of the reality about which we have in part fantasised and to which we have given the most beautiful colours. It throws us into a less agreeable reality that is no doubt closer to the truth. Maybe it becomes difficult then to emerge from one's 'cocooning' and accept the forgotten harshness of the world. But maybe it is important to surpass oneself every now and then in order to identify and change one's illusions. Is this one of the answers to our questions on the role of pain?

One can accept its paradoxes and, in this context, follow Kahlil Gibran's precept: 'Pain breaks the shell of one's ability to judge. Just as the stone must break for its germ to rise toward the sun, you must experience pain … It is the bitter medicine chosen by the doctor in you, to treat your diseased self.'

1 Merskey, H. IASP Sub-committee on taxonomy. *Pain terms: a list with definitions and notes on usage.* Pain, 1979; 6: 249-252.
2 Melzack, R and P.D. Wall. *Le Defi de la Dolour (The Challenge of Pain).* Maloine, Paris, 1982.
3 Freud, S. *Hemmung, Symptom und Angst,* 1926. Translated into French by Tort, M. *Inhibition, symptôme et angoisse (Inhibition, Symptom and Anxiety).* PUF, Paris, 1951.
4 There are cases of congenital insensitivity to pain which lead to an absence of nociceptive perception at the sensorial level. Children suffering from this disorder are constantly exposed to danger in the early years of their life. Piercing their own cheeks with a pencil, causing themselves to suffer bedsores and open wounds or burning themselves badly are some of the numerous examples of the mutilations they can suffer every day. It is necessary for these children to learn about the dangers of life in other ways than through the actual experience of pain.
5 Cyrulnik, B. Personal communication, 1991.
6 Le Clézio, J. M. G. *Le Jour où Beaumont fit connaissance avec sa douleur (The Day Beaumont Came Face to Face with His Pain).* Mercure de France, Paris, 1985.

Displayed Pain and
Hidden Pleasure

Jean-Didier Vincent

*'However, we say that we would not hesitate to express our gratitude
for any philosophical or psychological theory that could tell us what
is the real meaning of the sensations of pleasure and displeasure
which exert such an urgent action on us. This is the most obscure
and inaccessible area of psychical life. And since we cannot escape
its appeal, we think that the best we can do in this regard is to
formulate an hypothesis as vague and general as possible.'*

Sigmund Freud, *Beyond the Principle of Pleasure*

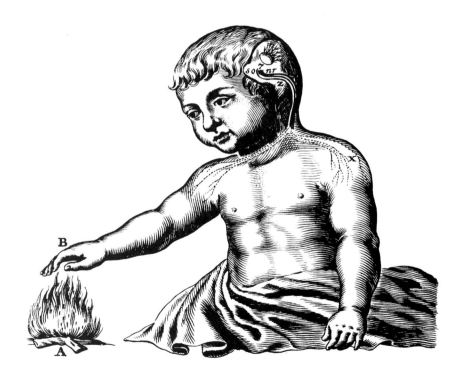

René Descartes. *Reflex Arch
(de Hominis Figuris, 1664).
(BIUM)*

EXHIBITIONS of pain attempt to make it a presentable object. Curiosity room and museum on the one hand, consulting room and hospital on the other, it is, in both cases, an attempt to reify suffering. From the medical point of view, we are taught about the itineraries, paths and molecules that the painful messages follow within the body. From the museum point of view, we are reminded of the fact that pain is also a spectacle.

Both these representations can be accepted, provided it is also acknowledged that, behind the object that is presented, there is a patient. Pain would not exist without someone to suffer. Next to this *real* pain, suffering offers itself for the others. The pain is either expressed or displayed in the form of a more or less noisy groan, from the inarticulated cry to the explicit speech or the diagrammatic representation, with gestures and mimics, expressing the drama within the body. Whether for oneself or for others, pain, with everything else this implies, belongs to the individual who is suffering in body and spirit.

The Subject of Pain

I cannot accept the distinction that is almost always made between real, organic pain believed to be the responsibility of the medical profession and imaginary pain which is, at best, the responsibility of the psychiatrist and the healer; as though the latter form of pain does not come from a real body, but from its ghostly double, devoid of all substance. And yet, as far as I know, there is no spirit without a body. It is the body that gives a spirit to the machine and not the reverse, as shown by the powerlessness of artificial intelligence – a product of computer science – when it comes to reproducing the slightest human feature by means other than misleading metaphors.

Organic or imaginary pains are located within cerebral representations. The representations are in past or present functional relationships with a world which is, in the first instance, the body of the subject: a set of components which belong to a hierarchical organisation represented in what is sometimes referred to as 'the image of the body'.

If I am speaking of the subject, it is in order to point out that the self is in an object relationship with the body. Since the concept of self tends to refer back to psychology only, I am going to use the term subject in the phenomenological sense, to refer to the *real being* which is part of the *being*.

Furthermore, the world is, through the body, an extraphysical world, a space which is indifferent or protective and which especially includes the 'others' with whom the subject can form a social body.

Whether it concerns the physical or the extraphysical, the world would not exist had there not been a brain to give it a representation. We do not have direct access to reality; we only have a perception of this reality through the channels of our sensations.

Finally, the world is spread out through temporality. It is this time that

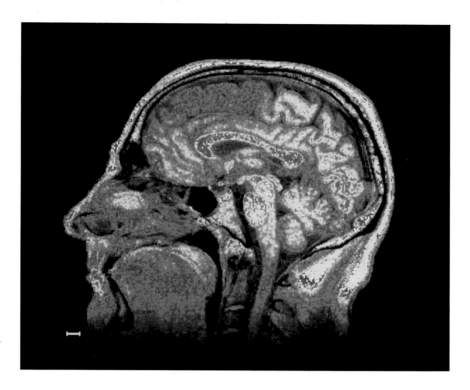

Brain. Imagery by Magnetic Resonance.
(CNRI)

makes the subject exist; for it is through the subject that it merges with temporality. As Merleau-Ponty put it: 'My body takes possession of time. It makes a past and a future exist for the present. My body is not a thing; it creates time and is not subjected to it.'

The Categories of Pain

In this context, pain seems to play its role: as an affection of the being. According to Szasz, a maximum of three categories of pain or levels of friction can be distinguished.

The first category is that of pain as a signal through which subjects record the fact that they are being threatened in terms of the actual integrity of their structure and function. This essentially concerns a modality of communication of subjects within their own body.

The second category affects beings in their relationship with others. One can, in this regard, speak of an emotion through which subjects let others know about the existence of a physical disorder for which they are seeking help. Any attempt to communicate the experience of pain to others leads to an exchange of meaning and, obviously, raises the issue of authentication. Individuals who are suffering from pain constitute the basis of the knowledge that subjects have of their bodies. Through the gesture and the cry, a newborn offers this other privileged person, the mother, a share of this knowledge. Hence, a child has in its possession a number of innate representations which allow it to initiate communication with the other. It can therefore be said that language emerges from this shared original pathos. All functionalist theories of language recognise that one cannot understand how it works unless one is capable of perceiving more than the objective things that the words denote. Intersubjectivity, or the exchange of emotions with the other, allows individuals to check the validity of their feelings with regard to the reality of their innate representations. This is the situation concerning pain and its figurative translation at the surface of the subject.

The third category concerns pain or suffering as a fundamental passion of the being. It includes the preceding categories but goes beyond the signal and the interpersonal communication to acquire an ontological significance. At this level, it becomes inseparable from its passionate opposite: that is to say, *pleasure*.

Pleasure and pain bear the mark of the limits of our being: the abyssal call of the original void beyond which pleasure and pain combine like the manifestations of a single body. Happiness and suffering are the branches of the same tree trunk called desire which is inscribed in the thick foliage of our neurons within the obscure forest of the brain.

One must guard against any dualist conception of pleasure and pain or of the life and death instincts (eros and thanatos). As the philosopher Grassi wrote: 'In different situations, the pleasure and pain of the same real being are interrelated, and it is only within this dialectic that reality manifests itself.'

Locating Pleasure and Pain

Without trying to duplicate the itineraries, paths and substances of pain which are discussed at length in this volume, I will limit myself to some biological data that are directly relevant to what I have to say. First of all, to remind us of the self-stimulation phenomenon of animals: in this instance, an animal presses relentlessly on a lever that sends stimulus to certain parts of its brain, particularly in the lateral regions of the hypothalamus. This is done regardless of the satisfaction of basic needs, as if the animal, above all, preferred the pleasure that it gets from the stimulation. These regions of the brain have been called 'centres' of pleasure. Neurosurgeons have been able to establish that the same thing happens with humans. Electric stimulation distributed over some parts of the brain can sometimes induce pleasure. The behaviour of self-stimulation does not have a specific goal and is removed from need as well as from satiation; it excites desire and pleasure to the same degree.

Opposed to pleasure, there are, in the brain, median nerve structures, the triggering of which can cause some effects contrary to those of the lateral structures. Pleasure and approach for the latter, but aversion, pain and escape

opposite page:
A. and P. Pollaiuolo. *Martyrdom of Saint Sebastian. (circa 1475).*
(London, National Gallery)

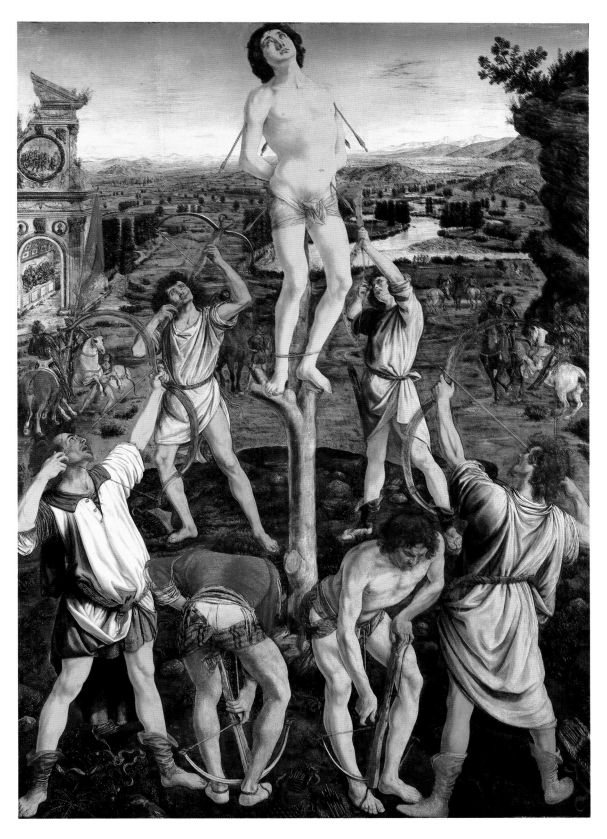

for the former. Pleasure and its opposite are nestled in a narrow area of the brain *that could be covered by the surface of a fingernail!* The reader might be shocked by this outrageous claim, that what supports the ontological basis of being is confined to ten grams of brain. But let everyone be reassured: as an 'open space', the hypothalamus is at the junction of everything that communicates within the brain, and no representation or act can escape its entry and exit visas. Finally, as a space with no specific location, the hypothalamus sums up the different components of subjectivity without locking them up in the centres.

Thus, the duality of pleasure and displeasure is reflected within the body itself by bringing into play the parasympathetic and orthosympathetic devices. Pleasure comes with a slowing down of the pulse and breathing, a fall in blood pressure, a contraction of the pupils, a salivation (to salivate with pleasure) and the secretion of various hormones, all of which are the general signs of parasympathetic activity. And yet, the brain centres which are designated as centres of pleasure and from which one gets self-stimulation also trigger parasympathetic activation. The reverse is achieved in the case of orthosympathetic suffering and activation. The affect is therefore inseparable from its physical dimensions. Unity of subjects in their being and appearance can be demonstrated even further by recalling Ekman's findings. These show that the parasympathetic and orthosympathetic translation of pleasure or pain can be measured in the body of an actor when asked to show these feelings.

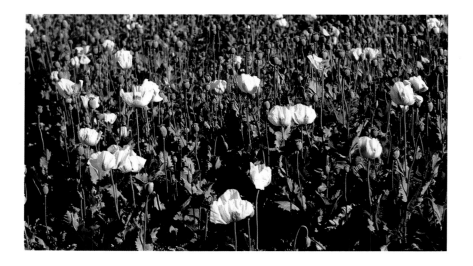

Field of Poppies. Drugs and the Brain.
S. Snyder, A.B. Joyce.
(Ph. Researchers Inc.)

The Opposing Processes

Not only do pleasure and suffering coexist in a corner of the hypothalamus, they confront one another in a constant embrace which is accounted for in the theory of opposing processes.

A striking example of these phenomena is that of the old story of the madman who is asked why he inflicts himself with hammer blows on the head and who answers: 'Because it feels so good when I stop!' Another example is that of the jogger who finds ineffable pleasure despite the daily torture on his legs and lungs. We know that quite often pleasure, when it is stopped, is paid back with intense suffering. The syndrome of deprivation experienced by drug addicts is a dramatic example of this. Opposites also coexist in our love life. Hence, the lover who cannot cope with the continuous happiness he enjoys with his mistress takes delight in the unhappiness of breaking off the relationship.

In addition to the syndrome of deprivation, two other phenomena are described within the context of the opposing processes: the affective contrast and the addiction or affective habit. An example of affective contrast can be seen in the state of distress created when a subject is brutally taken away from a source of pleasure. It is an object of imprinting in the case of a young bird and a transitional object in the case of a child (e.g. a blanket, a teddy bear). Imprinting is a strange phenomenon well known in the case of birds. It makes the newborn bird feel attached to a moving object which is presented at the time of hatching. When a duckling is deprived of the moving object that it has become attached to by imprinting, it becomes restless and shouts pitiful cries. On the contrary, addiction is the progressive disappearance of an affective state through repetition of the stimulus that created it. Repeated injections of morphine progressively lose their efficacy and a painful stimulus applied many times ends up not being felt any more. Affective contrast, addiction and the syndrome of deprivation are evidence of the existence of opposing processes. Hence, any factor responsible for a given affective state – pleasure or displeasure – seems, at the same time, to create a process of opposite direction in the body. This process develops with a certain degree of inertia and would seem progressively to oppose the first one. The consequence of both factors cancelling each other out would be at the origin of addiction. The opposing process is all the more evident when the affective factor is more intense and its repetition more frequent. When the affective factor stops, only the opposing effect remains in the form of a syndrome of deprivation or abstinence.

Addiction and abstinence immediately conjure up the idea of 'drugs': opium and its derivatives, morphine and heroin. Often focusing on the terrible opposing effects that they create, we tend too easily to forget the reason why they are used at all: pleasure. Opium is a good example of the negative relationship between pleasure and suffering. The same drug that suppresses suffering creates pleasure. Therein lies the trap into which the drug addict falls. Once the use of drugs ceases, there is nothing left but pain, a suffering

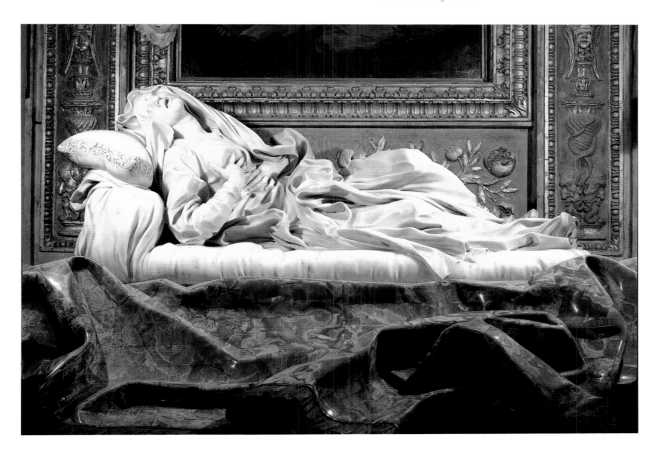

Bernini. The Blessed Ludovica
Albertoni. (Rome, St Francis Church)
(Cl. Artephot)

which has no meaning because it is deprived of pleasure and abandoned by morality. Should we therefore look for the origins of drugs in terms of suffering? Or should we leave to pain and pleasure the management of a homeostasis which is hopeless and only preoccupied with the survival of the species?

Pain and Knowledge

In avoiding the display of pain exclusively in terms of its neuronal and chemical aspects, I did not intend to overlook the fact that these make up the very substance of our passions. Rather, I wanted to show that suffering is part of the basic foundation of subjectivity. The painful feeling is only a component of the aversion one may have as a general manifestation of the being to the world. With regard to this aversion pain would play the primary role that some experiences of satisfaction play with regard to pleasure.

It is not my intention here to show how passions constitute the plinth on which the thought process is based (I do not want to use the scholarly term of cognitive functions), but again, simply to point out that pain is a way of gaining access to knowledge, and that this knowledge, in turn, plays a part in the

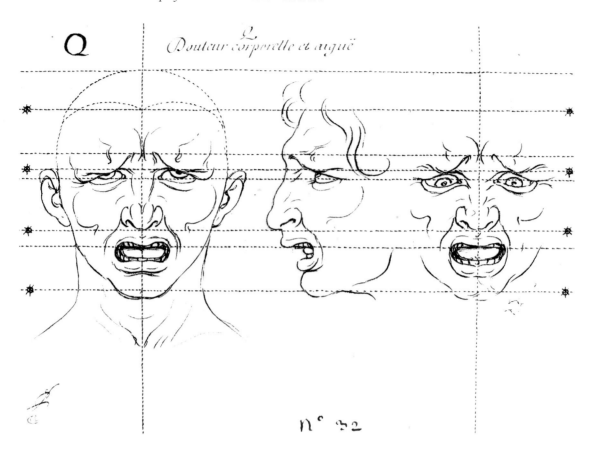

Q *(Douleur corporelle et aiguë*

n° 52

perception of pain. For instance, a painful stimulus will be perceived more or less strongly according to whether or not one knows about it ahead of time.

The real situations offered are never simple ones. No painful perception is pure and devoid of historical contingency. Any pain is perceived according to what surrounds and precedes it, sometimes very far in the past. Pain offers the possibility of tracing through the nerves the progressive transformation of a sensation into an affection. From the point of entry into the spinal cord, pain in fact collides with the descending flux of information coming from the brain, which modulates it by reducing or clarifying the message. At the level of the cerebral structures, the painful message mixes with the network of neurons which are responsible for the general processes of aversion and becomes an integral part of the desirous systems. If there still exist specific paths of pain that take over in the ventro-basic thalamus toward the somaesthetic cortex, these are no more than a fraction, sometimes negligible, of the evolution of pain which, from now on, finds its way through the limbo and the hemispheres.

Finally, it is true that, at a higher level, pain can come from representations in the brain with unnamed supports in which the comings and goings of the world have lost both their presence and actuality.

Charles le Brun (1619–1690). Study of facial appearance. Physical and acute pain. (Cl. Françoise Foliot)

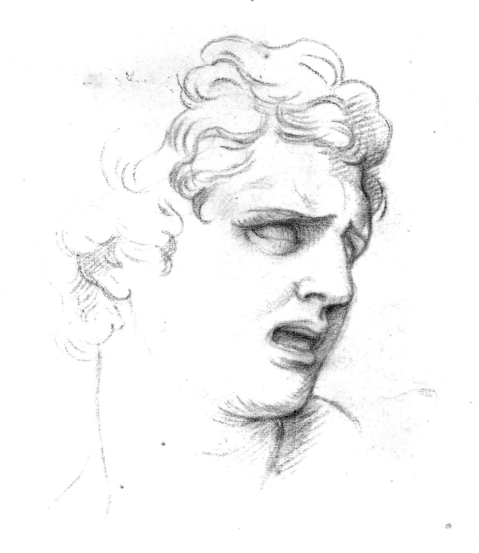

Charles le Brun *(1619–1690).*
Study of facial appearance. Acute pain.
(Cl. Françoise Foliot)

In Conclusion: On the Good Use of Pain

Pain is useful. It is the sign of a disorder somewhere in the body or of an injury suffered that should be stopped or healed. Veterinary surgeons know this quite well. This is why they sometimes hesitate to fit splints to certain fractures, leaving to pain the care of immobilising the animal much more rigorously than a splint would be able to.

The fact still remains that pain, as an element of actual experience, plays a critical role in the definition of the body. It means the conjunction of the physical and extraphysical spaces in which, according to Bergson 'the object to be perceived coincides with our body'.

The Christian world is based on the metaphysical and moral meaning of pain: this will be the only reference to a Passion whose biology escapes us. It is an important paradox that pain travels on the reassuring nerve pathways and the relays provided by the spinal cord as it communicates man's powerlessness and tragic history.

Should one take the side of pleasure against that of pain? It is true that Spinoza considers pain the most mediocre of passions. Pain says: go by and be done with! – but the Nietzschean hero sings: all happiness wants to last forever. The function of the opposing processes is to remind us that, during a party, waste and litter pile up.

Sacrifice, the ultimate meaning of pain, lights up stakes, activates bombs and crucifies gods. Is this suffering the inevitable result of the development of our brain? If the presence of a brain bathed in constraining secretions forces us to choose between pleasure and pain, why not choose the first as Pascal, Luther and Montaigne would have? It is a choice which is always jeopardised by the opposing processes, a choice that must be negotiated, a choice of courage and grace.

The Neurobiology of Pain

Allan I. Basbaum

ALTHOUGH most people have experienced pain at some time in their lives, the nature of the pain is usually limited in magnitude and duration. The pain of a broken leg or a headache can be quite severe, however the expectation is that the pain will resolve and that further treatment will not be necessary. Unfortunately, there are many situations in which pain persists, as for example, in patients with cancer or arthritis. Even more disturbing are situations in which pain persists in the absence of stimulation. One of the most striking examples of this is the phenomenon of phantom limb pain. Although all people who suffer an amputation of a limb will experience a phantom limb, a small percentage of these patients will not only experience the phantom, but will also experience severe pain in the phantom limb. Some patients may report that the nails of the fingers are digging into the hand of the phantom. A most disturbing aspect of this problem is that phantom limb pain is often unresponsive to traditional therapies for the relief of pain such as narcotics. In other cases, surgical intervention may have been attempted to relieve a particular pain and this may result in the replacement of the original pain by a new pain that is far more severe and disturbing. This type of pain, called neuropathic pain is typically characterised as severe burning. For example, pain can arise in an area of the body to which the nerves have been completely cut. That area of the body may be completely anaesthetic, yet the patient experiences severe pain in that region. This neuropathic pain, termed anaesthesia dolorosa, is extremely unpleasant, persistent and very difficult to treat.

To understand how such bizarre pain phenomena can arise, it is important to understand the basic anatomy and physiology of pathways which lead to the perception of pain. The key word here is perception. Pain is a complex perception that arises from the experience of an injury-producing, or potentially injury-producing, so-called noxious stimulus. Whether or not a given stimulus is perceived as painful depends not only on the intensity of the stimulus but

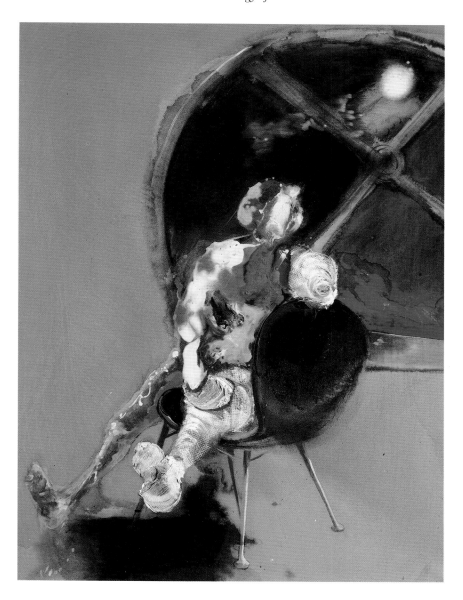

P. Rebeyrolle. *The Stump*
oil on canvas.
(Galerie Lelong)

on the immediate situation, on the past history and memories of the individual
and on the emotions that are generated by the stimulus. Not all injury stimuli
are perceived as painful. An athlete may receive a significant injury but not
experience pain until the match or event is over. Some women can deliver a
child with a remarkably small amount of pain if the birth experience is a
positive one; if not, it is likely that the pain experienced will be more severe.
Clearly, the intensity of the stimulus is not the only factor that determines
the magnitude of the pain experience.

Nociception: Transmission of the Injury Message

The process by which information about an injury stimulus is transmitted to the brain is termed 'nociception'. A classic view, articulated as far back as Descartes, held that there are specific pain pathways in the brain. It was proposed that once the particular pathway is activated, the perception of pain is the inevitable result. If specific pain pathways existed, it would be relatively simple for the neurosurgeon to interrupt the pathway and thus block the pain. It would be comparable to cutting a telephone line; the connection is always broken. Indeed, surgical attempts to block pain by cutting pathways have been made. Unfortunately, although sometimes successful, there are many instances in which persistent pain cannot be relieved by cutting a so-called 'pain' pathway. An examination of the elements within the nervous system that respond to noxious stimuli is critical to understanding why.

Our analysis begins in the periphery (e.g. in the arm, leg or face) where there are nerve fibres which respond to noxious stimuli. Nerve fibres in the periphery are of different diameters. The smallest diameter 'C' fibres (called nociceptors) conduct electrical impulses very slowly and are, in fact, selectively responsive to stimuli that usually provoke pain and which, if maintained, will cause tissue injury. Larger diameter 'A' fibres, by contrast, respond to non-injury-producing stimuli, such as brushing hairs or bending of joints. An important feature of the small-diameter nociceptors is that their threshold, though high under normal conditions, can drop precipitously, leading to situations in which stimuli that normally do not produce pain become very painful. This condition is referred to as hyperalgesia. Many people have experienced the pain of sunburn. In this case, stimuli such as light touch of the skin can provoke significant pain. Patients with arthritis report that the slightest movement of joints can be devastatingly painful. Hyperalgesia results from the lowering of the threshold for activation of the smallest nerve fibres in the periphery.

Hyperalgesia Mechanisms

Recent studies have provided considerable information about the mechanisms through which the threshold of small-diameter, 'C' fibres is lowered. When tissue is injured, there is a significant change in the chemistry of the membranes of cells. A product of this breakdown is the production of molecules called prostaglandins. When released from injured tissue, prostaglandins act upon the 'C' fibres and lower their thresholds for activation, so that stimuli normally not painful now produce significant pain. To treat this phenomenon, called *sensitisation*, one uses drugs that block the synthesis of prostaglandins. These drugs include aspirin and related non-steroidal anti-inflammatory drugs, NSAIDs, all of which are readily available. In fact, the majority of pain seen in clinics is of the hyperalgesic type and can be reduced, if not eliminated, by the use of this class of drugs. It is also possible to block the

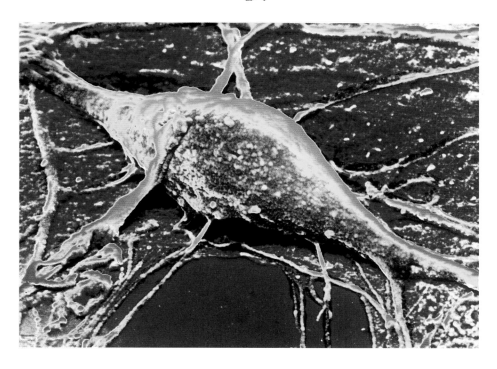

MEB Neurons. (Secchi-Lecaque,
Roussel-UCLAF) (CNRI)

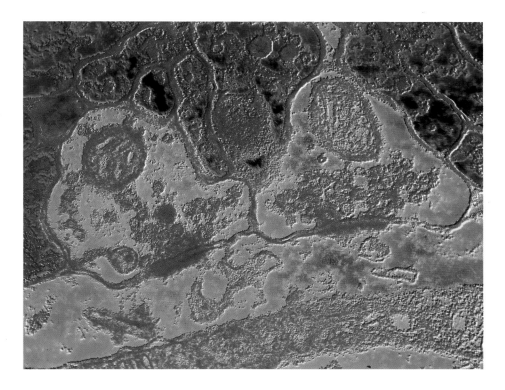

Synapses, axosomatic function.
(CNRI)

synthesis of prostaglandins using steroids. In fact, steroids are very effective for the treatment of the pain and inflammation of severe arthritis. Unfortunately, the side effects produced by steroids make them difficult to use for extended periods of time.

Transmission of the Nociceptive Message to the Spinal Cord

Nerve cells communicate by releasing chemical messengers that initiate electrical impulses in other cells. Information is thus transmitted along chains of nerve cells from the periphery into the central nervous system. Of great interest are recent studies that have identified molecules associated with the transmission of nociceptive messages from the peripheral nerves to the second order nerve cells in the spinal cord. In particular, the eleventh amino acid peptide, substance P, is a major player in this system. Substance P (the 'P' stands for powder, the form in which the molecule was isolated) is synthesised by small-diameter nociceptive fibres and it is then transported to the spinal cord where it can be released to act upon second order nerve cells that will transmit the nociceptive message to the brain. That substance P is indeed involved in the transmission of 'pain' messages is indicated by the observation that injection of substance P into the spinal cord of rats evokes behaviour similar to pain. Recently selective antagonists that block the central effects of substance P have been developed by pharmaceutical companies. It is hoped that their further characterisation will lead to new approaches to modifying the pain experience relatively early in the transmission pathway.

That this approach may prove helpful is indicated from the use of the molecule called capsaicin, the active ingredient in hot peppers. Capsaicin injected into the skin is very painful; indeed, the burning sensation produced by spicy food is produced by the capsaicin in it. A group of scientists from Hungary (the home of the capsaicin-containing paprika) found that when capsaicin is injected into neonatal rats (less than two days old), capsaicin acts as a neurotoxin. It destroys the small-diameter 'C' fibres that transmit nociceptive messages. The animal grows up with significantly reduced pain sensation, consistent with the loss of small-diameter nociceptors. In addition, there is a significant loss of the peptide substance P. Destruction of small-diameter fibres by capsaicin, however, is not an approach that one would recommend for the relief of pain in humans. On the other hand, repeated topical application of low concentrations of capsaicin in adult rats and in humans results in a dramatic desensitisation to subsequent noxious stimuli. That is, while initially producing pain, capsaicin subsequently blocks the ability of the small-diameter fibres to transmit information. In part, this is probably because capsaicin induces a depletion of substance P in these fibres, in this case without actually destroying the fibre. The trick is to develop a molecule that has the desensitising effects characteristic of capsaicin, but without its pain producing effect.

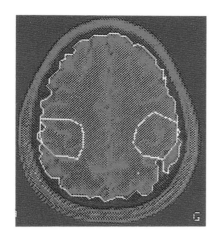
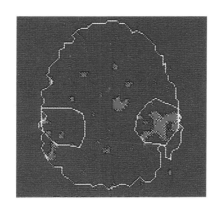
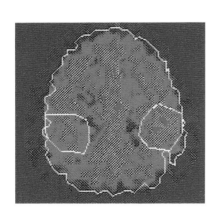
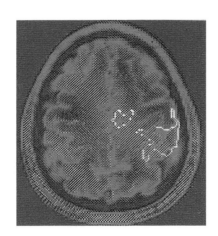

*Combined study in positron emission
tomography and magnetic resonance
imagery.
(Dr. Ph. Remy and R. Samson, F. Joliot
Hospital Service, DSV, CEA, Orsay)*

The Spinal Cord and its Connections
with the Brain

The specificity that characterises the responses of peripheral nerve fibres breaks down in the spinal cord, which is the first relay site for information transmitted from the different parts of the body. Although one can find some nerve cells in the spinal cord which respond relatively specifically to noxious stimuli, the vast majority can be excited by activity in both large-and small-diameter fibres, i.e. there is a convergence of information from non-noxious and noxious stimuli. This tells us immediately that whether or not a given stimulus is experienced as painful will depend on the activity of some fibres that do not respond to noxious stimuli at all. Indeed, there is evidence that activity in large-diameter fibres has the capacity to block the transmission of messages provoked by stimuli in small-diameter nociceptors. In fact people take advantage of this all the time. Imagine what happens when you burn your hand: typically you shake it. At first this seems like a strange thing to do. You have just massively stimulated your hand, for example, by burning it, yet to relieve the pain you stimulate it some more! Shaking your hand, or applying a vibrator, or using more sophisticated electronic devices called transcutaneous electrical nerve stimulators (a TENS unit), work because the stimuli selectively activate the large-diameter fibres. As indicated above, they have the capacity to block the firing of spinal cord neurons that normally transmit 'pain' messages. One can immediately see the difficulty that a neurosurgeon faces: how do you selectively cut spinal pain pathways when they do not exist?

Of course, there are pathways that transmit information from the spinal cord to higher centres in the brain and some of these carry information about the pain message. The problem is that they do not exclusively carry 'pain' information. In cases where all other therapies have failed and only in cases of terminal cancer where there is no hope that the patient will survive, the neuro-surgeon will cut all of the pathways associated with the transmission of the nociceptive messages, at the level of the spinal cord. This procedure is called anterolateral cordotomy and is used to eliminate the pain for the time the patient has to live.

In general, one can distinguish two major pain routes of information through which pain messages are transmitted. One is more involved in the localising aspect of the pain stimulus. That is, it provides information about the location of the injury. This pathway does not appear to access those parts of the brain which generate the affective or emotional features typically associ-ated with injury and clinical pain states. The second pathway from the spinal cord to the brain is much more diffuse and does not access these latter systems. It is likely that the transmission of information in the more diffuse pathway generates the qualities of pain that are typically associated with clinical pain states. Unfortunately, since they are so diffuse it is impossible for the surgeon to cut them selectively. Rather, it is necessary to use pharmacological

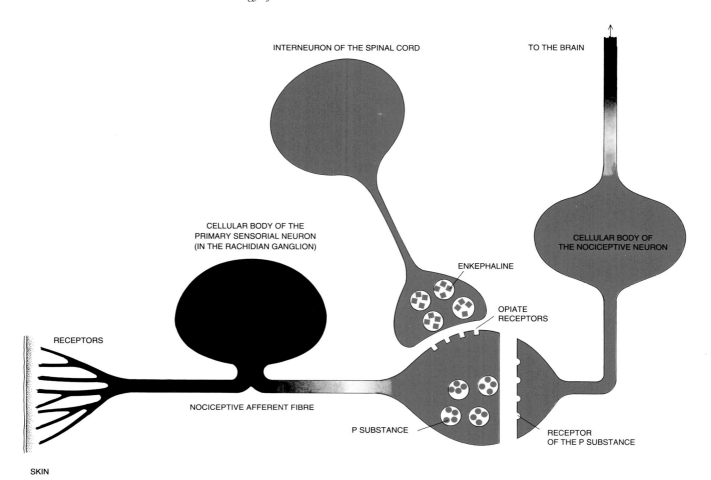

INTERNEURON OF THE SPINAL CORD

TO THE BRAIN

CELLULAR BODY OF THE
PRIMARY SENSORIAL NEURON
(IN THE RACHIDIAN GANGLION)

CELLULAR BODY OF
THE NOCICEPTIVE NEURON

ENKEPHALINE

OPIATE
RECEPTORS

RECEPTORS

NOCICEPTIVE AFFERENT FIBRE

P SUBSTANCE

RECEPTOR
OF THE P SUBSTANCE

SKIN

*Sketch of a control mechanism which regulates
the transmission of nociceptive messages before
the first synaptic relay in the spinal cord.
(P. Horber)*

approaches to the management of pain in order to block these very diffuse systems. The most effective therapy for severe pain involves the use of narcotics (i.e. morphine and related compounds).

The major target of the spinal cord pathways is the thalamus, a structure that relays information to the highest processing region of the brain, namely the cerebral cortex. One of the most important and as yet unanswered questions is where in the cortex pain is processed. Since pain cannot be elicted by electrical stimulation of the human cortex (in the conscious patient) and because it is difficult to eliminate pain by even large ablations of the cortex, it has, in fact, been proposed that the cortex is not necessary for pain perception. In my view, however, the complexity of the pain experience makes that possibility highly unlikely. Consider the analogy between pain and beauty. Although we have considerable information about the processing of visual information and know the areas of the cortex that are involved, we have little information about where the perception of beauty is processed in the cortex. Beauty is a perception that is 'coloured' by emotions and experience; it is an individual experience, much like pain. It may be the case that no one area of the cortex subserves the perception of pain.

A new approach to observing the activity of nerve cells in the human cortex has, however, provided exciting information about the different areas that may be involved. Called PET scanning, this approach involves sophisticated imaging methods and to date has identified regions of the cortex that are activated when humans experience pain. Such approaches will hopefully provide information that can be used clinically to monitor the experience of pain and to evaluate the mechanisms through which drugs that relieve pain – i.e. analgesics – modify the cortical response to injurious, pain-producing stimuli.

Pain Control Mechanisms

The observation that stimulation of large-diameter fibres has the capacity to block pain, or at least reduce it, was the basis of a very famous theory of pain published in 1965. This is referred to as the Gate Control Theory of Pain. Briefly, the theory argued that whether or not a stimulus is perceived as painful depends not only on the intensity of the stimulus but on the relative activity generated in large-and small-diameter primary afferent nerve fibres. It was proposed that there is a gating mechanism in the spinal cord. Activity in small-diameter 'C' fibre nociceptors 'opens the gate'; large-diameter fibre activity closes the gate by bringing in inhibitory mechanisms. In fact, there are many anecdotal observations that non-noxious stimulation in addition to shaking your hands, is effective for the relief of pain. As a general class these pain relieving approaches are referred to as counter-irritation mechanisms. Among the most interesting is acupuncture. Although traditional acupuncture suggests that stimulation of points along different meridia in the body can lead to regulation of pain at other sites of the body, the fact is that acupuncture needles are often administered in the region of the pain itself. That is, if your left arm hurts, the acupuncturist might needle the left arm. This may very well be a form of counter irritation, i.e. a form of gate control.

Non-segmental Pain Control Mechanisms: Opioid Analgesia

The relief of pain by non-noxious stimulation carried over large-diameter fibres is called segmental pain control. It is only exerted over that segment of the body where the pain originated: if your left arm hurts, you don't rub your right foot. It is also possible to produce much more global regulation of pain. This is particularly evident when one evaluates the mechanisms through which the narcotics produce their analgesic (i.e. pain-relieving) effects. Before discussing the mechanism through which narcotics exert their effect, however, it is of interest to describe a different form of analgesia, one which, it turns out, operates via very similar mechanism to that of the narcotics. In the late 1960s, it was reported that if an electrode was implanted in a particular part of the brain called the periaqueductal grey, and current was applied to the electrode, it was possible to render an animal completely pain free, without producing major side-effects. Soon after this observation was reported in animals, it was demonstrated that electrical brain stimulation could produce similar pain control in humans with chronic pain. Based on a variety of anatomical and physiological studies, it was confirmed that electrical brain stimulation works by turning on a very powerful inhibitory control system which blocks the transmission of 'pain' messages at the level of the spinal cord. In other words, the information from the periphery, i.e. from the site which receives the noxious stimulation, is no longer transmitted from the spinal cord to the brain. Pain control is the result.

Of particular interest is the observation that the analgesia produced by electrical brain stimulation can, under certain conditions, be reversed by the opiate antagonist, naloxone. That is, a drug that is typically used to block the analgesia produced by morphine and related compounds can block the analgesia produced by electrical brain stimulation. This led to the hypothesis that brain stimulation evokes the release of molecules that mimic the action of morphine. Indeed, it is now well documented that the brain contains chemical compounds, called endorphins, which have many properties similar to that of morphine. Endorphins are peptides, which although structurally quite different from morphine, act at similar sites in the brain to produce their effect. These sites, called the opiate receptors, are distributed in wide regions of the brain, including many areas that are involved in the transmission of 'pain' messages. Morphine exerts its effect by substituting for the endorphins. It has been proposed, therefore, that electrical brain stimulation produces analgesia by 'tapping' into the endorphin-mediated pain control system through which morphine operates. Naloxone, the opiate antagonist, blocks electrical brain stimulation because it interrupts the endorphins' action at the opiate receptor.

Other studies indicate that morphine can also block pain by acting directly at the level of the spinal cord. Small injections of morphine into the cerebrospinal fluid surrounding the spinal cord can produce very powerful and prolonged pain control in both animals and humans. This approach to pain control is now one of the most common approaches for post-operative pain. Direct spinal injection of morphine is also beginning to be used for chronic pain, as occurs in cancer patients. In these patients a pump is implanted near the spinal cord. This pump provides a continuous infusion of morphine at the level of the spinal cord. The great advantage of this approach is that there is a very selective block of pain transmission and limited side-effects. The side-effects, such as respiratory depression and euphoria, are much less common than if the drug were injected systemically, i.e. into a muscle or vein.

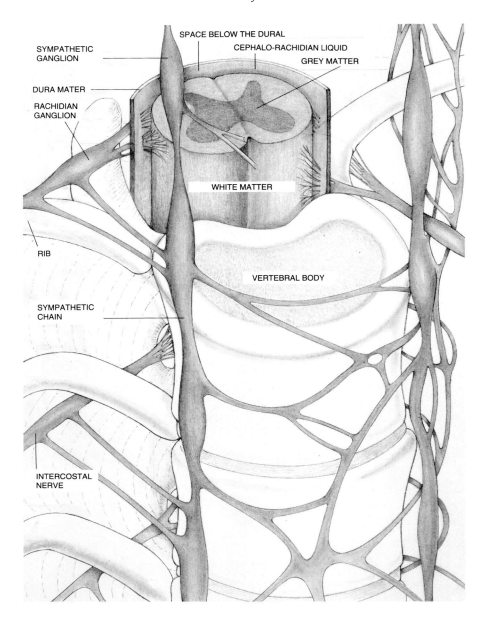

The spinal cord receives nerve fibres from the periphery of the organism and transmits the messages to the brain – it is immersed in the cephalo-rachidian liquid where the morphine is injected for the treatment of intractable pain. (P. Horber)

Alternative Approaches to Pain Control

There is an unfortunate common misconception that if a patient responds to a placebo, i.e. a psychological intervention, their pain must be imaginary. In fact studies suggest that the greater the injury, i.e. the greater the pain, the more likely the patient is to respond to a placebo. One of the more dramatic reports in recent years is that the analgesia produced by placebos can be reversed by naloxone. The fact that naloxone can antagonise some of the analgesia produced by placebos indicates that placebos have the capacity to access the endorphin-mediated pain control system. Understanding the means through which psychological factors can regulate pain is an important step in developing new methods of pain control.

Not all forms of pain control involve endorphin release. Thus, for example, one of the most powerful ways of blocking pain is through hypnosis. In this case, it appears that the pain message is transmitted from the periphery to the spinal cord and then to the brain, however, the perception that would normally be generated is altered in a completely unknown manner. Pain is not perceived as it would be if the hypnotic suggestion were not initiated. The development of the pain perception is presumably interrupted, at the level of the cortex. Consistent with hypnotic analgesia working differently from opiates, the analgesia produced under hypnosis is not sensitive to the opiate antagonist naloxone, indicating that endorphins are not involved.

In summary, it can be seen that we now have a remarkably detailed understanding of the physiological mechanisms that contribute to the transmission of the nociceptive message. Although we do not understand how the injury message is translated into a pain perception, many new approaches to interrupting the transmission pathway have been developed. These are certain to dramatically improve the care of patients with chronic pain.

Modern Strategies in the Development of New Analgesics: From Opium to Endogenous Opioids

Jean-Marie Besson and Bernard P. Roques

As one of our colleagues in pharmacology, the director of research of a major pharmaceutical industry laboratory, recently pointed out, the pharmaceutical industry cannot boast of its recent activities in the discovery of new analgesic substances. In fact, as early as the fourth century before Christ, Hippocrates was already mentioning some properties of the bark of the willow tree containing salicin, a compound of the acetylsalicylic acid (aspirin) family. This medication is still widely used in the world for the treatment of pain and fever. Likewise, the poppy, from which morphine was extracted until recently, was grown by the Sumerians 3000 years before Christ. It was not until much later, thanks to progress in chemistry, that the active principle in these plants was isolated. Morphine was not isolated until 1806. A large number of active principles from plants or those secreted by micro-organisms (a good example of this is penicillin) constitute the basis of our pharmacopoeia today.

It is therefore not surprising that the discovery of medicines has been essentially due to chance, but also to the persistence and observing minds of researchers and clinicians. To illustrate this last case, in the field of pain, some antiepileptics and antidepressants are used today to try to suppress particular types of pain, notably pain arising from lesions of the peripheral and central nervous system. Here again, the use of these substances does not result from rational research, but simply from accidental observations by some particularly attentive clinicians. In France, although a few hundred pharmaceutical products are classified as analgesics, they are frequently analogues of the same molecules. In fact, there is only a small number of original molecules, some of which have a moderate analgesic activity (e.g. aspirin, paracetamol and other non-steroidal anti-inflammatory medicines), whereas others, particularly morphine or its derivatives, have an extremely powerful effect and, when prescribed following strict rules, can, in most cases, suppress intense pain of cancerous origin (in 70% to 90% of cases, according to research).

Twenty-five years ago, chemists synthesised molecules, essentially taking into account the physico-chemical structure of those which were isolated from plants. The toxicity of these molecules was then assessed with different classical tests, and their possible physiological and pharmacological properties were finally assessed *in vivo*, mainly on rodents. It was therefore tedious and slow research requiring a large number of animals and the results of which, as we have already indicated, were mostly due to chance.

However, research in the field of pain has expanded considerably during the last twenty-five years, especially after the discovery of opioid receptors and endogenous substances made and released by some cells of the nervous system and with some properties akin to those of morphine.

The receptors are molecules which are located on the surface of nerve cells. Morphine or endogenous opioids specifically bind to these sites and bring about a chain of biochemical reactions which lead to pharmacological effects. Hence, with various biochemical techniques, it is now possible to quickly specify the number of receptor sites and the affinity (the binding force) for a newly synthesised substance for a given receptor type. As for morphine and its derivatives, there is a good correlation between their affinity for the receptors

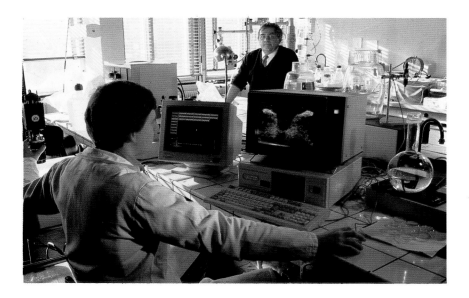

The laboratory of physiopharmacology of the nervous system of Inserm, headed by J.M. Besson (in the background), is one of the main research centres on pain in France. The analgesic role of morphine at the level of the receptors located in the spinal cord (shown here on the screen) was discovered at this research centre.
(Ph. Plailly)

and their pharmacological activity. These techniques can be used on brain slices, allowing a rapid selection of substances according to the strength of their action. One can therefore quickly analyse the effects of certain molecules on a very small number of animals, and it is only after this first screening that the most promising molecules are studied *in vivo* on different animal species, particularly rodents. These binding techniques have been extended to the entire field of pharmacological research, especially in the area of neuroscience. In other words, we have moved from empiricism to rationalism.

As pointed out by Allan Basbaum in his paper on the neurobiology of pain, there are several directions of research concerning the pharmacology of pain. The aim of this research is to develop the ideal analgesic; i.e., a substance which has the power of morphine, but which lacks undesirable side-effects (e.g. addiction, dependence, respiratory depression, constipation). There are various experimental strategies that are not just concerned with developing products acting on the opiate receptors. Aspirin, for example, has an effect mainly at the peripheral level, and modulates the excitability of the numerous nerve endings located in the skin, the muscles, the joints and the viscera. But aspirin also produces undesirable side-effects, particularly through its direct action on the stomach mucous membrane. Here again, a new drug acting with the same mechanism, but without these disadvantages, would undoubtedly have a therapeutic future. This is also true for other substances called monoamines, especially noradrenaline and serotonin. These substances are contained in nerve cells located in the lower part of the brain and send messages in the direction of the spinal cord, in order to inhibit the transfer of nociceptive messages at this level.

Many research groups are trying to develop selective agonists; i.e. substances which can imitate the activity of natural molecules by acting on receptors that are specifically involved in the control of pain. However, although several tens of thousands of molecules have been synthesised as possible analgesics, there has been a series of disappointments because, among other things, pharmacology is confronted with the multiplicity of receptors. In fact, for the same monoamine or peptide, there can be several types or sub-types of receptors, which with the techniques of molecular biology have been well characterised.

Understanding pain means, first of all, trying to comprehend its physiological mechanisms. When the nervous system is not damaged, its tracts, relays and information centres are relatively well defined, even though there are several unknowns with regard to the mechanisms involved in the brain itself. Numerous cerebral structures are involved in the different components of pain (i.e. sensory-discriminative, affective and emotional, cognitive) of this highly subjective phenomenon which remains quite difficult to quantify. The problem, alas, is even more complex in the case of pain caused by lesions of the nervous system, whether this is of a peripheral origin (e.g. damage to the medullary roots in motorcycle accidents, AIDS-related, diabetic or alcoholic

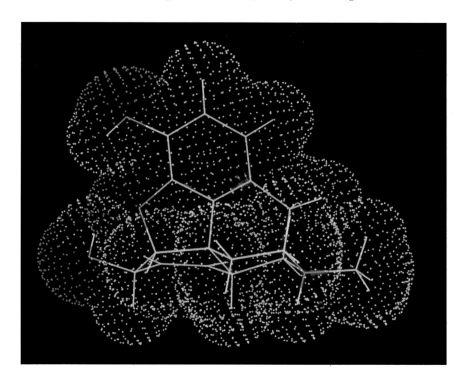

A morphine molecule. (Ph. J.C. Revy)

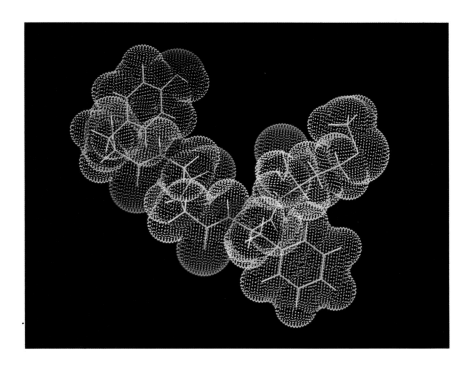

*Molecular modelisation of a molecule of
enkephalin – Atomic skeleton plus Van der
Waals envelope. (Ph. J.C. Revy)*

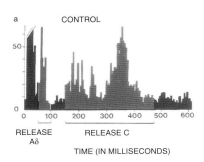

a   CONTROL

RELEASE
A δ   RELEASE C

TIME (IN MILLISECONDS)

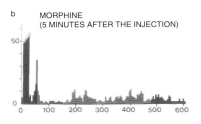

b   MORPHINE
(5 MINUTES AFTER THE INJECTION)

TIME (IN MILLISECONDS)

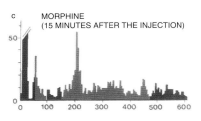

c   MORPHINE
(15 MINUTES AFTER THE INJECTION)

TIME (IN MILLISECONDS)

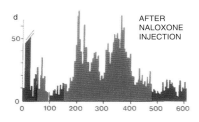

d   AFTER
NALOXONE
INJECTION

TIME (IN MILLISECONDS)

neuropathies) or of a central origin (e.g. lesion of the spinal cord, vascular cerebral accidents). These types of pain are often very difficult to relieve. The pain is present without any stimulation. Some of them are permanent and stubborn, whereas others are sudden and are similar to the pain felt in cases of serious burns or electrical shocks. They are complex syndromes whose physiopathological mechanisms are difficult to identify. To tackle these problems, the main research teams working in this area at the international level have attempted to experimentally simulate pain in rats. Obviously, the development of such models is limited by ethical regulations. But as long as these are observed, and as long as the researchers follow the accepted procedures set down by the ethical committees supervising this type of research, the importance of such experiments justifies this undertaking. The major models used (e.g. acute or chronic inflammation, rheumatoid arthritis, moderate compression of the peripheral nerve) do not produce all the painful syndromes that are seen in the clinics. However, they yield some new data with regard to the physiological, behavioural and pharmacological aspects of pain.

More recent visualisation techniques, which are starting to produce spectacular advances in this area, should be added to the various multidisciplinary approaches that have been developed, in order to try to decipher the different aspects of the psychopharmacological puzzle of pain. This is the case with the use of the positron camera in humans, and that of proto-oncogenes (cancer genes which, in the absence of any pathology, are involved in the normal operation of cells) as an index of the metabolic activities in animals during painful events.

In the midst of these various approaches, we are probably heading towards a new understanding of the mechanisms of the different types of chronic pain, and therefore, towards a more rational development of the appropriate therapeutic approach.

The uncertain nature of the therapeutic research pointed out at the beginning of this paper is mainly due to the dearth of information on the structure of natural molecules such as endogenous opioids and their receptors as well as their receptor mechanisms. This makes any attempt to develop a tailor-made substance capable of imitating (agonist) or blocking (antagonist) the effect of a natural messenger very difficult.

The considerable progress achieved during the last fifteen years in the field of molecular biology and in the definition of chemical structures has led to significant advances in therapeutic research. For example pain must first of all be considered as part of the information which enables a living organism to set off avoidance strategies in order to preserve its integrity (e.g. the sudden withdrawal of a hand inadvertently placed on a burning surface). Pain passes through specific tracts where endogenous opioids and opiate receptors are located, so that it is not confused with the tactile sensation, for instance. The binding of endogenous opioids (especially the enkephalins) and opiate receptors reduces the feeling of pain and therefore sets an acceptable threshold

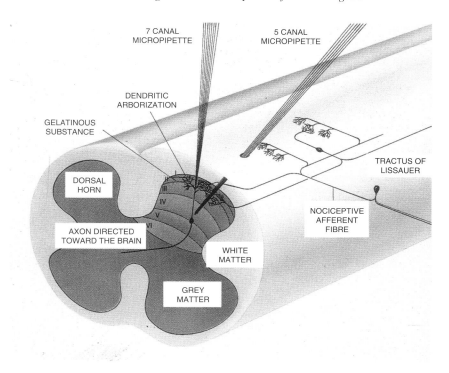

Effect of morphine at the level of the spinal cord, 5 minutes after the injection. (Fidia-France, Electra)

which is low enough for the organism not to suffer any injury, and high enough for it to avoid getting confused with the sensations (such as tactile) which are inevitably associated with every action.

This physiological control of pain could however be overwhelmed by violent stimuli at the skin level (cuts and burns) as well as at the nerve level (necrosis of a dental nerve) or at the visceral level (perforation of a stomach ulcer). In all of these cases, the stimuli cause the release from the damaged tissue, of algogenic substances such as two small peptides (bradykinin and substance P) which also settle on specific receptors located on the pain nerve endings.

Several strategies are currently used to produce analgesics which may be as potent as morphine but which lack the harmful side-effects mentioned above. One of these strategies consists in preventing the algogenic substances from acting on their receptors by means of molecules which can roughly be compared to keys fitting a specific lock (the receptor) but which cannot turn inside the lock and so cannot 'open the door in order to let pain in'.

These antagonists of bradykinin or of substance P can now be obtained by making use of the precise structure of the natural molecule. This is done by analysing the diffraction on an X-ray beamed on each atom or by decoding the peaks corresponding to the absorption of energy of each atom (most often an

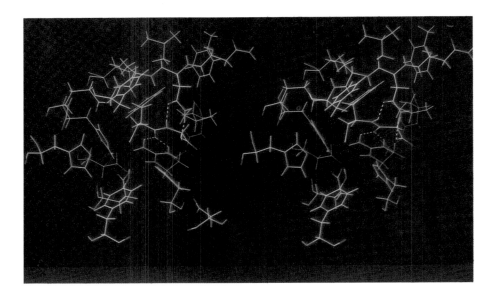

A representation by molecular modelisation of two inhibitors within the active centre of the neutral endopeptidase (on the left, the retrothirphan, on the right, the thiorphan). The orange dots show the hydrogen liaisons between the inhibitor and the enzyme.
(Fidia-France, Electra)

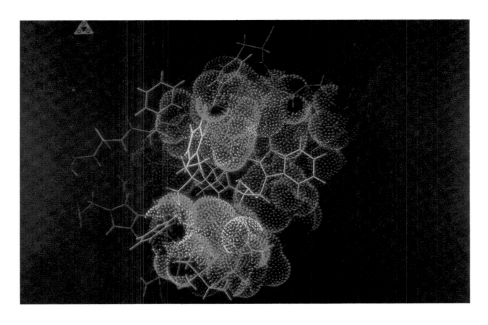

Docking of an inhibitor within the active centre of an enzyme by molecular modelisation.
(Fidia-France, Electra)

atom of hydrogen) using an instrument of nuclear magnetic resonance (NMR). A very precise representation of the molecule is then obtained, and this representation can be 'visualised' on a television screen. Since the receptors are at least one hundred times larger than their messengers, very few of them have as yet been analysed with the same precision. However, their primary sequence, i.e., their amino acid sequence which is obtained from the data of molecular biology (cloning), can be compared, thanks to computer techniques. Models can be developed in which it will be possible, again with computer techniques, to simulate the manner in which the chemically synthesised antagonist interacts with the receptor. These experiments known as 'docking' are used more and more, in order to guide the chemical synthesis.

The second rational approach has the advantage of being 'physiological'. It is based on the fact that endogenous opioids are released in small quantities from the nerve cells involved in the control of pain, located in the spinal cord and in the brain. The endogenous opioids are quickly destroyed by two enzymes. The active centre of these enzymes is very well characterised, the site where the binding of the most important endogenous opioids, the enkephalin occurs. Molecules (inhibitors) which bind in the active centres of these enzymes have thus been synthesised and prevent the enkephalins from gaining access to the centres. An increase in the concentration of the enkephalins follows and elevates the pain threshold by their binding to the receptors for the opiate morphine solutions. There are many advantages in using these inhibitor molecules instead of morphine. Their effect is limited to the areas

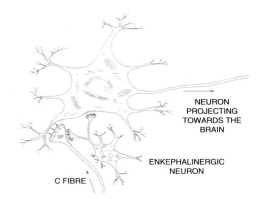

*Mechanism of the possible actions of morphine
at the medullar level.
(Fidia-France, Electra)*

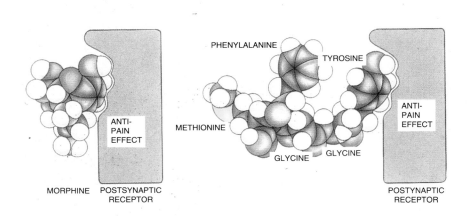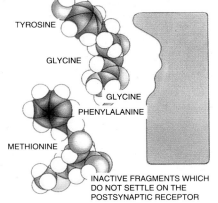

*Sketch representation of morphine molecules,
of methionine-enkephalin, and of the
degradation of methionine-enkephalin
in the central nervous system.
(Fidia-France, Electra)*

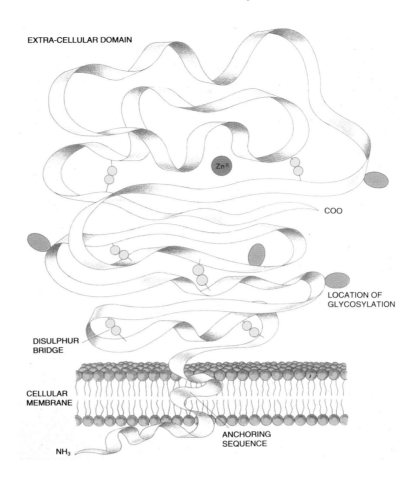

EXTRA-CELLULAR DOMAIN

Zn^{II}

COO

LOCATION OF
GLYCOSYLATION

DISULPHUR
BRIDGE

CELLULAR
MEMBRANE

ANCHORING
SEQUENCE

NH$_3$

Diagram of the structure
of neutral endopeptidase.
(Fidia-France, Electra)

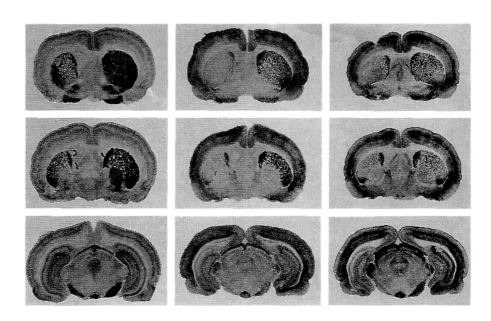

Three sections of the brain of a rat comparing
the distribution of neutral endopeptidase
(left column), of the delta opiate receptors
(right column) and of the opiate receptors
(centre column).
(Fidia-France, Electra)

where the enkephalins are released, whereas morphine 'floods' all the opiate receptors without discrimination. The limited effect of the molecules produces very little or no side-effects (tolerance, dependence, constipation). Their only disadvantages are that, firstly, their analgesic strength is somewhat lower than that of morphine and, secondly, they lack a certain degree of selection with regard to the enzymes.

This concept of 'physiological analgesia', which from the chemical point of view has greatly benefited from some modern techniques, from now on must be backed up by clinical tests. This is also true for the development and the use of opiate based agonists which selectively activate one receptor. It was found that in the spinal cord, the stimulation of the delta opiate receptors results in an analgesia almost as good as that induced by morphine by acting on *mu* receptors; but the responses are independent, additive and lacking in cross tolerence. Pain which has become resistant to morphine would then be reduced by the delta agonists. Here again, the first clinical results are expected with great anticipation.

In conclusion, we are fifteen years from the discovery of the natural control systems of pain by endogenous opioids. This may seem like a very long time before one can benefit from a therapeutic application, but it must be borne in mind that new directions of research involved in the development of new drugs are rare. It is difficult to compete with morphine for its analgesic efficacy; but, theoretically, this is a challenge that can be won. The most important thing is to fill some of the gaps in the treatment of pain using substances which have no side-effects, even after long-term treatment.

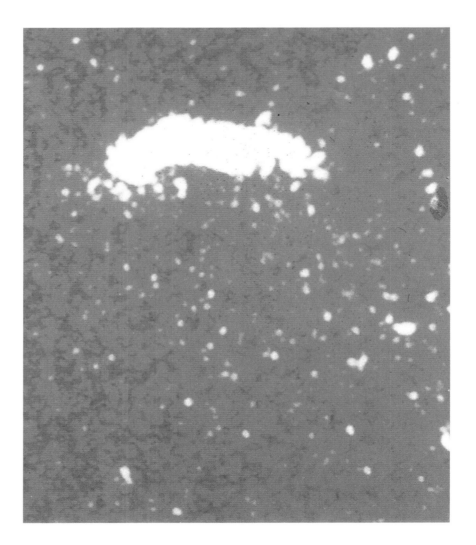

Localisation of neutral endopeptidase in the
dorsal horn of the spinal cord.

The Neurosurgeon and Pain

Jan Gybels

Faced with the failure of the medical treatment of intractable, intolerable and chronic pain, the physician may consider resorting to a neurosurgical operation with analgesic consequences.

For many, surgery means the surgeon's knife. But in fact, the needle, the catheter and the electrode have often replaced the knife in the operating theatre.

The concept of pain surgery has evolved considerably over the last few years, thanks to technological and scientific progress. Open surgery has now given way to the introduction of electrodes through the skin under local anaesthesia or general anaesthesia of short duration. This procedure also allows the doctor to verify the exact location of the nerve tracts involved in the transmission of the nociceptive messages (i.e. the reception of harmful stimuli). The introduction of an operating microscope helps identify the subtle compression exerted by some vessels on the cranial nerves which causes paroxysmal neuralgia, such as trigeminal neuralgia (generally known as *tic douloureux.)* This can be treated by elimination of the nerve tracts under specific conditions.

Techniques of Destruction of Nerve Tracts Carrying Nociceptive Information (Technique of Provoked Lesions)

Initially based on the knowledge of anatomy, the neurosurgery of pain was necessarily a surgery of lesions. But it was soon realised that 'pain often runs in front of the surgeon's knife': the nervous system has the remarkable capacity of regenerating itself to its pre-lesion state and of developing mechanisms that are little used or new and, therefore, of making the initial pain reappear at a later stage, or else, of activating an entirely new kind of pain classified as 'disafferentation pain'. And for this reason, surgery that will destroy a nerve tract is often no longer advised.

49

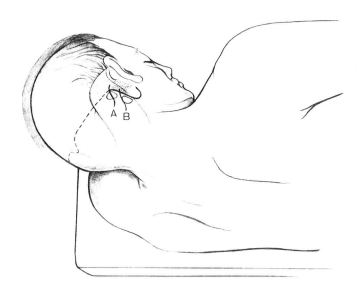

*Compression. Illustrated Techniques
in Microneurosurgery.
H. Kikuchi and A. Hakuba (eds),
1990, p. 260. Igaku-Shoin*

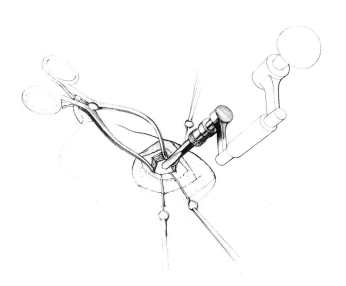

*Compression. Illustrated Techniques
in Microsurgery.
H. Kikuchi and A. Hakuba (eds),
1990, p. 261. Igaku-Shoin*

However, a major indication is represented by the intractable trigeminal neuralgia mentioned above. Here one can resort to percutaneous thermocoagulation of the Gasserian ganglion. According to this technique which was developed in the early 1960s, a percutaneous puncture is performed just next to the labial commisure, and an electrode is introduced through the natural hole located at the base of the skull, in order to reach the Gasserian ganglion. This ganglion is a structure in which the neurons responsible for the innervation of the face are located. The position of the electrode is checked by electrical stimulation and the ganglion is heated up to 80 degrees centigrade by way of a high frequency source of electricity. Generally the absence of painful crises in the face lasts for a while. However, there may be side effects such as disorders of limited sensitivity in the affected branches of the trifurcating nerve related to the pain.

As for pain in phantom limbs as a result of amputation or the avulsion of the brachial plexus (which is often the result of a motorbike accident), one can create a lesion which is mainly directed either toward the radiculomedullary junction or the dorsal horn of the spinal cord. In the 1970s, neuroanatomical studies of the penetration of the posterior root in the spinal cord showed that, with human beings, the small amyelinated fibres (C fibres) are distributed to lie in front of the large myelinated fibres (A fibres), which condition sense of touch. Thus, it is possible, through a microsurgical procedure, to achieve analgesia while preserving sensitivity to touch.

Furthermore, neurophysiological studies have underlined the fact that at the time of an accidental lesion leading to the removal of the roots, the neurons of the dorsal horn acquire some special properties which create a focus of

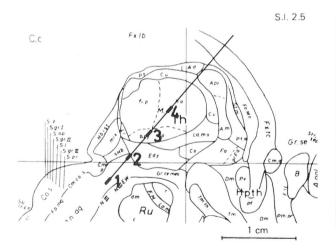
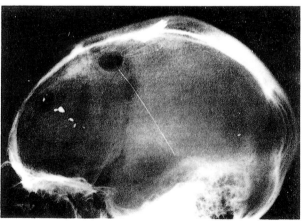

Electrode in the Gasserian ganglion.
Neurosurgical Treatment of Persistent Pain.
J.M. Gybels, W.H. Sweet, 1989,
p. 308. (Karger)

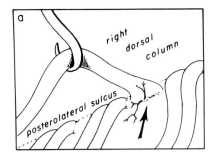

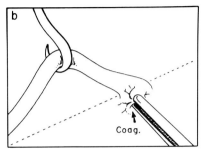

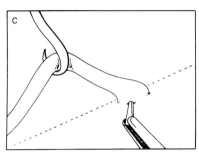

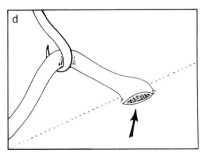

Radicellectomy. Neurosurgical Treatment of Persistent Pain. J.M. Gybels, W.H. Sweet 1989. p. 129. (Karger)

irritation at this level. In the 1980s, some procedures, known as dorsal root entry zone or DREZ were developed with a view to destroying, generally through small lesions induced by electrocoagulation, the foci of abnormal activity partly responsible for pain in phantom limbs.

Anterolateral cordotomy should also be mentioned here for historical reasons. Developed at the beginning of this century, it was one of the first neurosurgical operations performed to treat serious and persistent pain which resisted any other form of treatment. It was one of the most frequently used operations, especially in the case of pain due to cancer. Its objective was to block the nerve tracts transmitting the nociceptive information located in the frontolateral region of the spinal cord. Since the 1960s, this operation has been performed under local anaesthesia by puncture at the high cervical level of the spinal cord under radiological monitoring and with neurophysiological location of the target. The localisation process can be very complex. This procedure contributed significantly to the body of knowledge on the organisation of the spinal cord in human beings. It was also very successful until the mid-1970s. Toward the end of the 1960s, new neurophysiological techniques considered conservative (in the sense that they leave the nervous system intact) slowly replaced the techniques of lesion described above. These new techniques are known as neuromodulation.

These 'conservative' techniques are based on recent findings regarding the neuroelectrical and neurochemical control mechanisms operating in nociception; these findings are described in other contributions to this volume. They are also the result of data obtained from patients suffering from chronic pain. Clinicians have taken advantage of these ideas in activating the inhibiting controls of nociception, with a therapeutic goal in mind.

The advantages of neuromodulation techniques are twofold: their efficiency can be tested before the final operation, and they are perfectly reversible and do not have any adverse side-effects.

These new 'conservative' techniques, i.e. neuromodulation, comprise two major sectors: electrical neurostimulation with an analgesic objective and intrathecal morphinotherapy.

Electrical Neurostimulation with an Analgesic Objective

According to the pathology, surgery by electrical neurostimulation can be performed at three different locations which, from the periphery to the centre are the following: the peripheral nerves, the posterior spinal cord and a number of nuclei of the thalamus.

The positioning of the active electrode depends on the area one desires to stimulate. The choice of this area depends upon the kind of pain and its distribution: for peripheral nerves, the electrode, which is shaped like a ring, is directly inserted by open surgery on the peripheral nerve corresponding to the painful region; for the spinal cord, the electrode, which can be of various

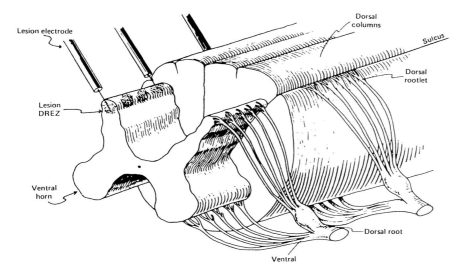

DREZ – dorsal root entry zone. Journal of Neurosurgery, 51, 59–69 (1979).

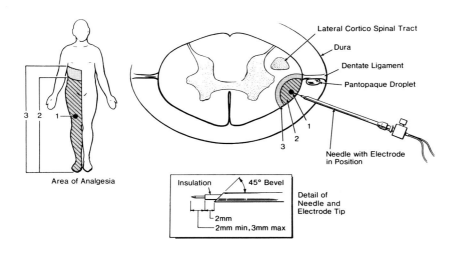

Set-up for cordotomy. IASP Refresher Courses on Pain Management, 1990, p. 131. IASP Publications, Seattle.

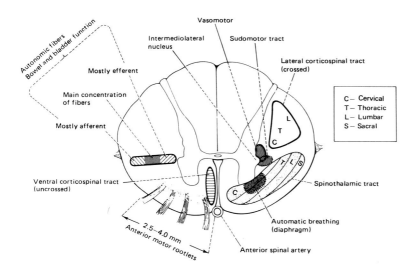

Functions within the spine. Neurosurgical Treatment of Persistent Pain. J.M. Gybels, W.H. Sweet 1989. p. 164. (Karger)

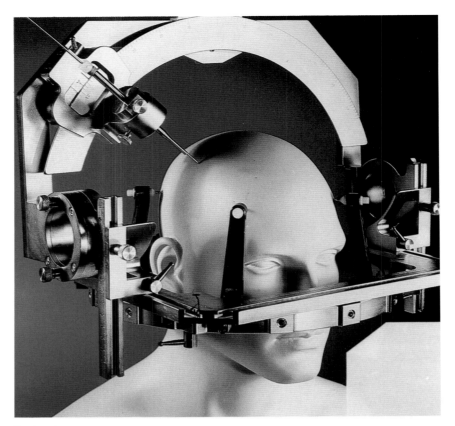

Steriotaxie.

shapes, is introduced in the posterior epidural space. In most cases, this is performed by way of percutaneous penetration, just like a lumbar puncture. In some cases, a laminectomy, i.e., the removal of a small part of the posterior arch of a vertebra, may be necessary; for deep cerebral stimulation, especially that of the thalamus, one must resort to a specialised technique of stereotaxis for the insertion of the electrode. This technique is based on the principle that a point can be defined in space, provided that the co-ordinates of the three lines which meet through this point are known.

If activation of the electrode, which is connected to an external stimulator, effectively stops the patient's pain, an internal stimulator is then implanted. This is necessary because a direct external connection between an electrode and a stimulator would expose the patient to serious risk of infection. In addition, such a method would be uncomfortable for the patient and aesthetically not acceptable. There is a variety of models of stimulators that can be implanted.

In one type of stimulator only the electrode and the radio frequency receiver are implanted. The external part of the system, which is given to the patient, comprises a radio frequency transmitter which allows a modulation of the signal and which is connected to an antenna fixed on the patient's skin next to the transmitter. Thus, the patient chooses the different parameters of stimulation.

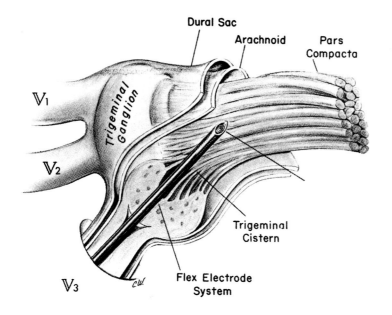

Electrode on the spinal cord.

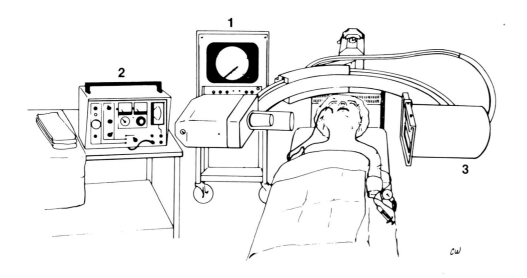

Stereotaxis. Operative Neurosurgical Techniques, Vol. II. H.H. Schmidek, W.H. Sweet (eds). 1988. p. 1112. (W.B. Saunders)

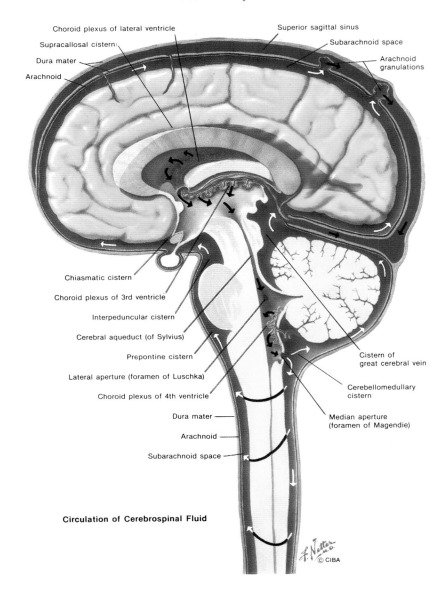

Circulation of Cerebrospinal Fluid

Ventricles and area of circulation of the cerebrospinal fluid. © Copyright 1986 Ciba-Geigy Corporation. Reprinted with permission from The Ciba Collection of Medical Illustrations, illustrated by Frank H. Netter, MD. All rights reserved.

The other category of stimulators are those which can be totally implanted. The energy source of the impulse generator is part of the device. These systems, which are more comfortable for the patient, are programmed telemetrically by the physician. The patient can start or stop the device with a magnet.

Clinical experience has shown that the best indication for neurostimulation is chronic pain caused by a lesion in some part of the nervous system (disafferentation pain). It is well known that this pain is resistant to other types of analgesic treatment such as medication, methods of psychological inspiration, physiotherapy, etc. Causes include traumatic lesions of nerves, phantom limbs, development of cicatricial tissue after the removal of a slipped disk, which leads to the constriction of root lesions to the spinal cord due to an accident and lesions to the brain following a stroke.

Administration of Morphine in the Spinal Fluid

The cerebrospinal fluid present in the space which surrounds the brain and the spinal cord (the intrathecal space) has been used for a long time for the administration of local anaesthetics and other substances in the treatment of pain. But an interest in this area and in the ventricles located within the brain (which are in communication with the intrathecal space and also filled with cerebrospinal fluid) was triggered by the discovery of neurons in the spinal cord and the brain which have receptors that bind with opioids.

After this discovery, it was soon realised that intrathecal injection of morphine and other opium-based drugs can provide a strong analgesic effect without affecting other sensations, interfering with motor activity or producing addiction or sedation. Hence, localised morphinotherapy, especially at the level of the spinal cord, in the intrathecal space, and when necessary, at the cerebral level in the ventricles, developed rapidly. This conservative and totally reversible procedure is almost exclusively used nowadays for the treatment of chronic and intractable pain of malignant origin. To a large extent, it has replaced cordotomy.

Localised morphinotherapy is performed by implanting a reservoir in the body under the skin, often at the level of the abdomen. The morphine is introduced into the cerebrospinal fluid through a catheter.

As for the types of 'reservoirs' two options are currently possible.

One method uses a small reservoir equipped with a self-sealing membrane, which is placed under the skin and allows for repeated subcutaneous punctures. This system replaces the puncture made in the intrathecal space (lumbar puncture) with a simple subcutaneous puncture which administers the appropriate dose of morphine. This system is suitable for short term treatment.

The second method, using implanted pumps which have ten or twenty times the capacity of the reservoir mentioned in the first method, allows the patient a reserve of medicine and more autonomy. Depending on the level of sophistication (and also the price) of the device, one can have flexible

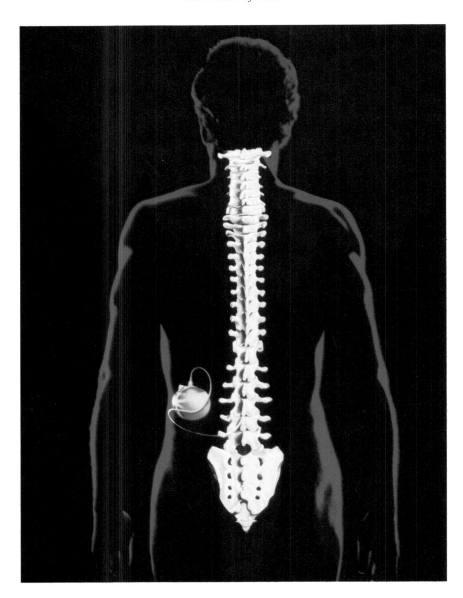

Programmable morphine pump. IASP
Refresher Courses on Cancer Pain, 1990.
IASP Publications, Seattle.

schedules of repeated, continuous or repeated and continuous release of fixed doses of a given drug.

Intrathecal morphinotherapy is therefore used in cases of otherwise irreducible pain resulting from cancer. The important prerequisite selection criteria are as follows: significant reduction of pain during intrathecal injections on a trial basis; a favourable environment allowing for the follow up of this treatment as an outpatient; the consent of both the patient and the family after adequate explanation; the possibility of managing the potential side-effects of the intrathecal administration of morphine with an implanted device.

The possible side-effects are: a respiratory depression, itching sensations, urinary retention, bouts of nausea and vomiting, and morphine tolerance.

Some Concluding Remarks

First, it is important to note that neurosurgery as a means of treating chronic pain is justified only after the failure of medical treatment (medical in the sense of 'non-surgical'). After medical treatment has failed and the patient continues to suffer, neurosurgical techniques, some of which are very sophisticated, can be resorted to in order to control the pain. It is up to the physician to choose the most appropriate technique for a given patient; i.e., the technique which, in a specific case, is the most efficient, the least dangerous, the cheapest and the most comfortable. When faced with a difficult choice, it is useful to remember that the pain we endure best is the pain suffered by others.

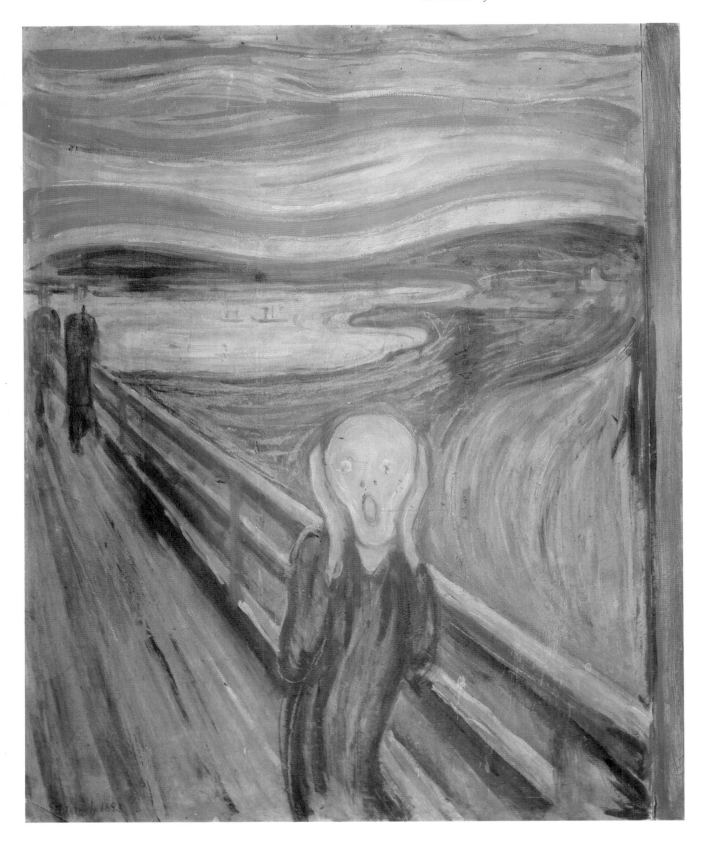

Pain Treatment Centres

François Boureau

PAIN is a daily and commonplace experience. In most cases, it is a transitional episode which terminates favourably. However, with some patients, pain will persist, resisting treatment and becoming chronic. The public is often misinformed on this possibility.

Little research has been done on the proportion of the general population that suffers from chronic pain. Nevertheless, the available data show the importance of the phenomenon. Taking a period of more than 100 days over the past year as a criterion, the NUPRIN report found that headaches affect 5% of the general population, back pain 9%, muscular pain 5% and pain of the joints 10%.

Acute and Chronic Pain

It has become very common to distinguish between acute pain, an alarm system symptom, and chronic pain, a complete illness with a trail of psychosocial factors. Chronic pain refers to daily pain which has been developing over six months. A number of differences in the neurophysiology, the neuropsychology and in behaviour justify the distinction made between acute and chronic pain. Regardless of its initial etiology, chronic pain cannot be perceived only as persistent acute pain.

Diversity of the physiopathological mechanisms

To put it simply, there are three types of pain: nociceptive pain, neurogenic pain and psychogenic pain.

Pain caused by an excess of nociception

Pain is most often a symptom, an alarm signal of injury to tissue, resulting from trauma or pathology which must be diagnosed. The mechanism in question

opposite page:
***E. Munch.** The Cry.*
(Oslo National Gallery)
(Ph. Giraudon)

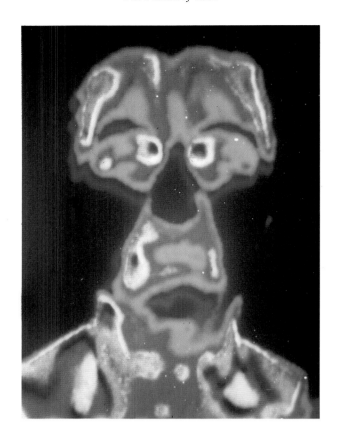

Migraine before the crisis (thermography). (G. Ravily) (CNRI)

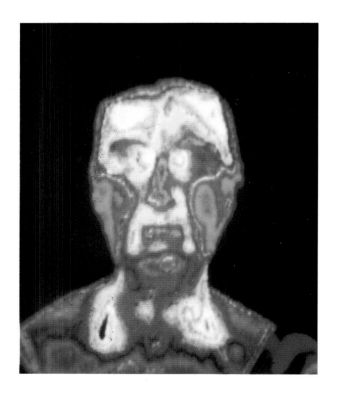

Migraine during the crisis (thermography). (G. Ravily) (CNRI)

is an excess of nociceptive stimulation. At the level of the centre of the lesion, the peripheral nociceptors are stimulated mechanically and/or by various algogenic substances. The transmission system of nociceptive messages is therefore needed in its periphery. The treatment for a slipped disk or a tumorous exeresis will be etiological as much as possible. At the level of symptomatic treatment, peripheral analgesics, anti-inflammatory non-steroidals and narcotics are resorted to, including techniques for the functional or anatomical interruption of the transmission pathways of nociceptive messages (i.e. anaesthetic blocks).

Excessive nociceptive stimulation is usually the reason for most acute pain. At the chronic stage, this excess is found in cases of persistent pathologies caused by a lesion. This is the case for chronic rheumatic or cancerous pathologies.

Neurogenic pain

Neurogenic pain is very different from pain caused by an excess of nociception, and was labelled deafferentation pain for a long time.

The underlying idea was that pain is mainly the result of the interruption of the afferents pathway (i.e., of the sensitive pathways) and not of their stimulation. The mechanism of deafferentation is probably essential to the cause of neurogenic pain; however, it is now acknowledged that peripheral mechanisms are also involved. Deafferentation remains the best example of a central

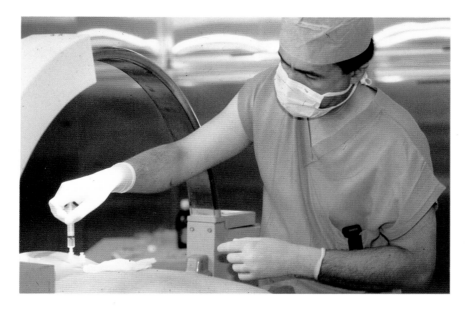

Centre for the Treatment of Pain,
Lariboisiere Hospital.
(Centre de l'Image – AP-HP)

mechanism generating pain. After a lesion or the interruption of peripheral pathways, the neurons of the spinal and supraspinal relays can become over-excited by mechanisms that are not yet fully understood. The main causes of neurogenic pain are phantom limb, post-herpetic neuralgia, a nerve lesion and paraplegia. These types of pain have the same clinical characteristics: anaesthesia dolorosa, which occurs in a totally insensitive area; allodynia which is caused by stimulation that is not painful under normal circumstances (e.g. the light touch of clothes); paroxysmal pain, which manifests itself in the form of sudden excesses of pain, similar to electric shocks. In the case of deafferentation pain, it is useless and illogical to prescribe peripheral analgesics or anti-inflammatory drugs. On the other hand, first-line medical treatment, such as the use of tricyclic antidepressants and anticonvulsants for the paroxysmal component, are of prime importance. Likewise, neurostimulation techniques are proposed whereas neurosurgical or anaesthesiological techniques, which can make the deafferentation worse, are rejected.

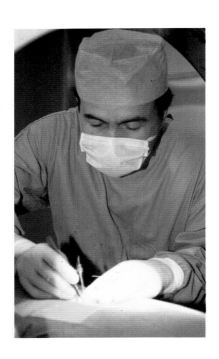

Centre for the Treatment of Pain,
Lariboisiere Hospital.
(Centre de l'Image.– AP-HP)

The psychogenic origin

Even though it's 'sine materia' nature could be suspected early in the scenario, it is often at the chronic stage that the 'psychogenic' origin of pain is finally considered.

Admittedly, the diagnosis of psychogenic pain is primarily arrived at when clinical and paraclinical investigations are negative. But this does not mean that it has to be a diagnosis of elimination. The psychogenic origin must be based on a positive psychopathological semiology. Various nosographic contexts that are part of the register of anxiety and depression are relevant.

Pain as a symptom and pain as a syndrome

Any pain, whether acute or chronic, is complex, multidimensional and determined by numerous interacting variables, some of which are: the sensory-discriminative, the affective and emotional, and the cognitive and behavioural. The sensory-discriminative component corresponds to neurophysiological mechanisms which allow the decoding of the quality, duration, intensity and localisation of nociceptive messages. The affective and emotional component expresses the more or less painful and disagreeable tonality which comes with any kind of pain; here, we return to notions of anxiety and depression. The cognitive component concerns the mental processes which can modulate the painful perception. These processes can attract or divert attention, change the significance, anticipation and expectations of pain, and refer to experiences of pain one has witnessed or suffered in the past. The behavioural component includes the manifestations of mobility (mimicry, restlessness or prostration) and verbal manifestations of pain (moaning and groaning), as well as all the repercussions in the various realms of activity of the individual.

Patients suffering from chronic pain are not a homogeneous population. Various physical and/or cognitive and behavioural factors may be implied.

The 'mixed' situation is the one most often encountered. The difficulty is that, for each case, the contribution of the various possible factors must be evaluated.

When pain persists, clinical investigation cannot bypass the evaluation of psychological and behavioural factors which are the causes and/or consequences of pain. The psychological consequences of persistent pain are often misunderstood and underestimated. Their role, as a factor of maintenance or during exacerbation of an originally organic pathology , must also be taken into account.

The health history of patients suffering from chronic pain is often illustrative. After several months of its development, patients suffering from chronic pain have generally seen many doctors. Their unsuccessful medical 'door to door' consultation maintains them in a passive state of resignation and hopelessness. Feelings of invalidity and social and professional inability dominate the patient. The painful complaint and the behavioural repercussions seem exaggerated in relation to the somatic data. Attempts by the doctor to recommend a psychiatric consultation are often perceived as a total lack of understanding of the pain (but my pain is very real, it's not imaginary!).

In order to understand and treat chronic pain better, doctors need to know how to analyse the various psychosocial factors which may take an interactive part in any kind of chronic pain, whether in a private practice or working within a multidisciplinary team. Thus, the effects of these factors go far beyond a simple diagnosis of psychogenic pain.

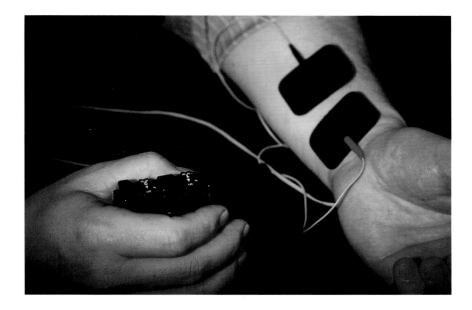

Subcutaneous neurostimulation device, located
on the median nerve. Prescribed method for
pain following a lesion to the nerve.
(ph. Plailly)

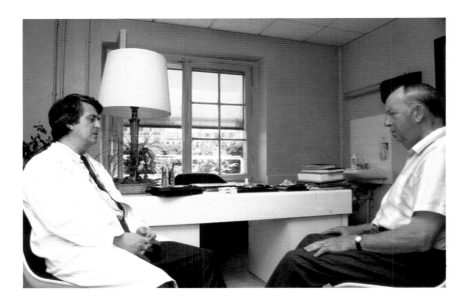

An anti-pain consultation, Tarnier Hospital.
A personal interview.
(Centre de l'Image – AP-HP)

Organisational Principles of Centres for Pain Treatment

The diversity of the mechanisms in question with regard to pain, the interactions with psychological and behavioural factors, and the multiplicity of therapeutic means currently available all help us understand that patients suffering from chronic pain need to be in the care of a trained multidisciplinary team.

In order to treat patients suffering from chronic pain, a large variety of structures can be envisaged. Organisational strategies must take into consideration the kind of pathologies examined, the range of proposed technical modalities and the nature of the facility (outpatient consultation or in patient accommodation). The problem lies in the ability to organise, at the same location and at the same time, co-ordinated procedures for the evaluation and the treatment of these patients.

Patients in centres for the treatment of pain are those who, in spite of an apparently correct medical diagnosis, at least at the somatic level, still continue to suffer from persistent pain which remains intractable to classical treatment. Chronic pain can be subdivided into two distinct categories: cancer pain and non-malignant chronic pain sometimes incorrectly labelled 'benign' pain. Their respective conditions of treatment are not comparable. Non-malignant chronic pain, is most commonly pain of the musculoskeletal system (post-surgical lumbo-sciatalgia), neurological pain, cephalgia and psychogenic pain. Cancer is a progressive ailment requiring continuous treatment which can become necessary at every stage of the illness. The treatment of pain cannot be totally separated from that of cancerous illness either; the problem at hand is not just limited to the terminal phase. Cancerous pain can benefit from a specific therapeutic arsenal: such as narcotics that are taken orally or injected, anaesthetic blocks and neurosurgical operations.

The principle of a multidisciplinary organisation is accepted these days, in order to better treat patients suffering from chronic pain. Beyond the juxtaposition of the disciplines represented, it is hoped that each team member benefits from the group contact, in order to synthesise an approach that could be called interdisciplinary or transdisciplinary. For the evaluation of patients, it becomes possible to go beyond the classic psychosomatic dichotomy, in order to integrate the totality of the somatic and psychosocial factors. The assessment is made in a multidisciplinary perspective of complementarity and not one in which reciprocal exclusion of the various factors of importance occurs.

The resulting therapy is therefore often multimodal and combines many techniques. One tries to propose treatments with etiological objectives as much as possible; but one also has to know when to resort to less specific approaches such as symptomatic, rehabilitative and psychobehavioural (e.g. relaxation and cognitive approaches).

Usually, the team must bring together specialists in the disciplines appro-

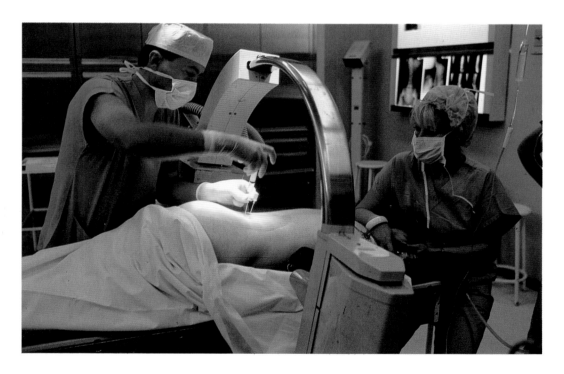

Centre for the Treatment of Pain,
Treatment of chronic lumbar pain: rhizolysis.
Lariboisiere Hospital. (SIPA Press)

priate for the analysis of the painful symptomatology under examination: a neurologist, a neurosurgeon, an anaesthetist, a rheumatologist, a physician, a psychologist and a psychiatrist.

Many other health care specialists are essential for the smooth and efficient operation of the centre: a nurse, physiotherapist and social worker.

The purpose of a centre for the treatment of pain is to gather together the most complete range of pharmacological, psychological, anaesthesiological and neurological techniques. The emphasis placed upon technical expertise must be balanced by a desire to use the techniques in the appropriate circumstances and to integrate them within a rigorous therapeutic approach. A good mastery of medical techniques will often relativise the focus sometimes put on medical expertise. It is important that, in each case, the therapeutic approaches envisaged are appropriate to the data of the medical and psychosocial evaluation. The therapeutic problems are different depending on whether or not one has a treatment with an etiological objective at one's disposal or at least a treatment which guarantees a strong possibility of relief.

Let us mention, for example, the importance of thermocoagulation for essential neuralgia of the trigeminal nerve, or a splanchnic block in cancerous pancreatic pain which is resistant to morphine treatment. It is in fact possible

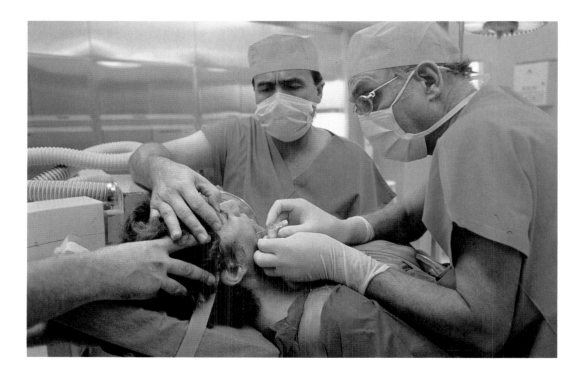

Thermocoagulation. Centre for the Treatment of Pain, Lariboisiere Hospital.
(SIPA Press)

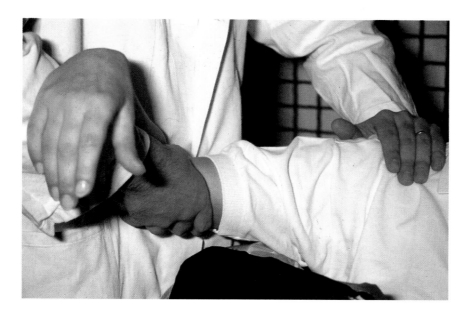

Centre for physiotherapy rehabilitation.
Corentin Celton Hospital.
(Centre de l'Image – AP-HP)

that the more specific a role a technique has in a generally accepted treatment programme, the more the concerned disciplines will use it widely without having to resort to a pain treatment centre. We are not going to provide an exhaustive list of the existing therapeutics of pain here. What is important to point out is the combined use of some techniques in the form of a therapeutic programme which implies a perfect co-ordination of the medical team. In addition, the process of providing care includes general non-specific medical attitudes which largely contribute to the results (explanations of the chronic pain and the attitudes one needs to adopt, approaching the patient regarding rehabilitation, reduction of the handicap, as well as family and professional reintegration).

The realistic objective is often to teach the patient 'to live with pain' so that it remains under control and does not become incapacitating. It is for such difficult cases that pain treatment centres play a specific role. This therapeutic follow-up unquestionably requires practical experience.

Conclusion

The creation of pain treatment centres is a step that will probably lead to an in-depth analysis of an area which has at times been neglected. Their role is not only one of evaluation and treatment of patients who are suffering from pain, but also one of clinical research, teaching and dissemination of the current information on pain.

In any event, one must remember that there is not just one but many kinds of pain and that progress achieved in one area cannot necessarily be transferred and applied to other forms of pain. Progress in this area is conditioned not only by the development of efficient techniques, but also, and most importantly, by the use of these techniques in the appropriate clinical context.

Physical Pain in the Middle Ages

Georges Duby

HISTORIANS nowadays are constantly extending their field of research. A few years ago, death was the subject of thorough and fruitful studies. As a result, historians have turned their attention not only to the body and its experiences, but also to the importance people attached to their bodies in the past. The history of what they ate, what they wore, of their medical practices, the history of plagues and starvations as well as the history of medicine – long put aside in France – are coming back into prominence. However, historians have not yet taken interest in physical pain. And yet, pain clearly does have its own history. The way it is perceived and the role it plays within the value system has evolved through time. We can see that these vary from culture to culture. They also vary through space. These variations no doubt deserve a close analysis in the global history of sensibility. I would therefore like to see research focus on the history of pain. For the time being, and in so far as the period I have some knowledge of is concerned – i.e. the feudal era, a truly rich period between the year 1000 and the beginning of the thirteenth century – I can only make a contribution to this new line of research by offering a few superficial remarks I have been able to draw from a prolonged study of the documents available.

These documents are scattered. Most of what one would like to learn about this era is obscure and within these sparse documents reference to pain is rare. The culture to which I am referring, a feudal culture dominated by priests and warlords, seemed unconcerned with physical pain; or at least, it was less anxious about it than our own culture. This is the impression we get from reading the documents accessible to us; that is to say, the feelings and the thoughts of the 'intellectuals' of that time, most of whom were members of the upper classes of the Church hierarchy, and who are the only ones to have left written or tangible evidence of their ideas and reactions. Pain was rarely talked about, rarely mentioned in the discourses of the time. This indifference to, or suppression of, pain raises a problem. But in accounting for it, it would be too

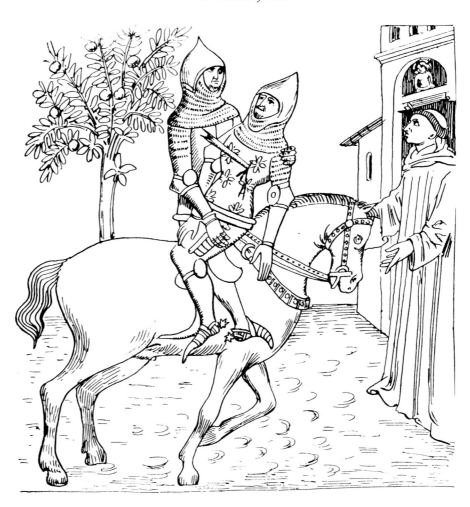

Wounded knight taken to a monastery for care. (Roman de Lancelot du Lac – Bibliothèque Nationale) (Centre de l'Image – AP-HP)

simplistic to explain it away only in terms of the primitive customs, the barbarity, and the heavier bearing of nature on the lives of primitive people whose living conditions, until the middle of the twelfth century, had apparently not changed much since the neolithic age; a people who were barely protected against cold and starvation and of whom one might therefore think as hardened against pain. It is already more advantageous to refer to the fundamentally male and militaristic characteristics of the ideology that prevailed back then. This ideology relegated women to a position of total subordination while it dignified the male virtues of aggression and tenacious resistance to attack. Hence, there was a tendency to hide all weaknesses and not to show compassion for physical lapses. Nevertheless, it seems possible to go even further in the interpretation of these documents.

The Latin vocabulary often used by the intellectuals of that time may be revealing here. An almost complete synonymy was in fact established between the word *dolor* or pain and the word *labor* which meant work. This semantic equivalence sheds light on the perception of physical pain in a value system

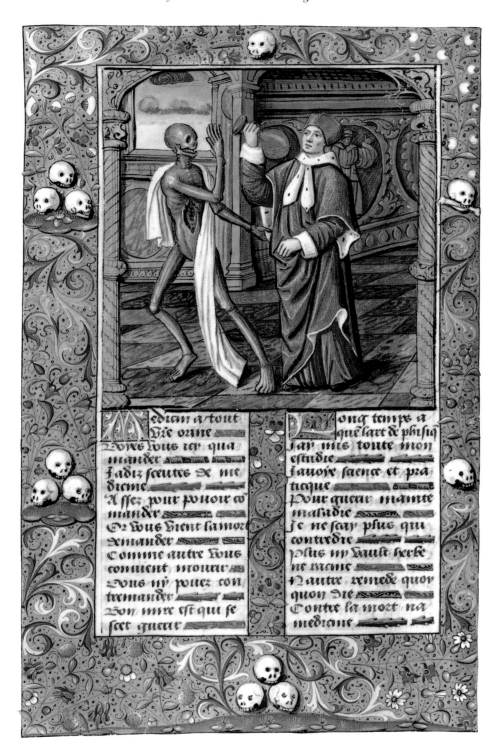

Danse Macabre.
(Bibliothèque Nationale)

that was based on two major foundations: firstly the Bible; secondly, the remains of the moral treatises of classical antiquity.

In the Judeo-Christian tradition, pain was perceived and presented as a test and as a punishment inflicted in anger by God. For instance, the Almighty overwhelms Job to test him, but he thrashes Israel. He begins by punishing Adam and Eve for their disobedience. This is how everything starts, with our first parents and their mistake. Man and woman are doomed not only to die but also to suffer, for having been led into temptation. But the woman will especially suffer from *dolor* – 'You shall give birth and experience pain' – and the man will especially suffer from *labor* – 'You shall earn your living by the sweat of your brow'. The punishment is a deserved one. Men and women are natural sinners. Therefore, it is quite normal that they should suffer. It is not only normal, it is also necessary that they should suffer. Hence, isn't it going against God's will when one tries to escape pain? Isn't it questioning the order established by the Creator himself? We all know too well that such mental representations have not been totally dispelled today.

As a result, pain is first and foremost a female matter that men must therefore hold in contempt. A real man does not suffer. In any event, he must not show any sign of suffering, for fear of losing his virility or being brought down to the level of the female condition. But it also follows from this that, because physical pain is associated with the idea of work, it seems particularly unworthy of a man who is not in bondage. The Greco-Roman tradition reinforced this attitude since it identified freedom with leisure and considered servile any form of manual work. Pain, like manual work, was therefore considered a fall from grace in the feudal era. It was thought of as a form of enslavement, and this further restrained priests and warlords – the only men to be truly free, because they belonged to the two functional categories superior to that of the workers or the serfs – from showing any sign of pain.

Such a conception is clearly reflected in the way crimes were punished: only those of a lower class, women, children, the obedient peasantry were liable for physical punishment whereas the members of the ruling class were only made to pay fines, and not subjected to the physical pain which would have tarnished their reputation and dignity.

Punishment was of the sin, and thus a sign of the sin; it was a sign also of enslavement and therefore a degrading one. As a result, pain only took on a positive value as an instrument of punishment, of atonement and of redemption. On one hand, this explains the place assigned to pain in the hereafter, an institution which took shape at the end of the twelfth century, and in purgatory (which left men with a thorny question: How could a soul separated from the body endure physical pain?). On the other hand, it also explains the place assigned to it in those other instruments of penance, the monasteries. The monks forced macerations upon themselves by humiliation in the same way that they undertook manual work.

It is therefore with regard to souls in purgatory and ascetics, that evidence

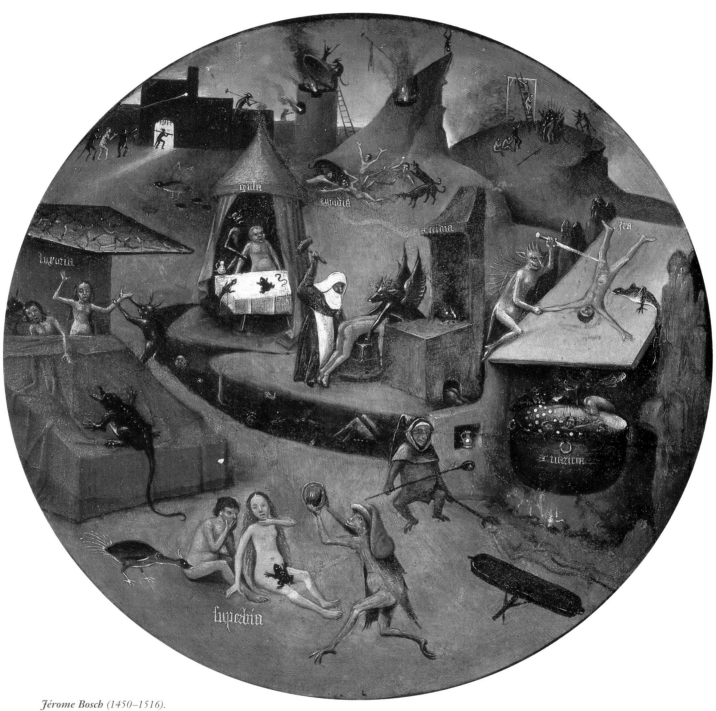

Jérome Bosch (1450–1516).
The Seven Deadly Sins. Detail: Hell.
(Madrid, Prado Museum).
(Cl. Giraudon)

abounds in texts and pictures that the historian of pain can use. As a matter of fact, it is almost the only available evidence. The literature which offers more information on what would nowadays be regarded as medicine, namely the collections of miracles, does not concern itself with physical pain, except when it reports on punitive miracles, the ones carried out by insulted saints who took their revenge by tormenting their offenders. But in the miracles of healing, references to pain are generally omitted. Most of these miracles are in fact similar to those that Jesus accomplished: they are about blindness, paralysis and being possessed by an evil spirit, ailments that are not particularly painful. As for chronicles, descriptions of battles or disasters, they are in relation to the tribulations of the human body; they describe injuries and frightful mutilations, but these descriptions are always made without any sign of emotion. It was as though the victim of these cruelties did not feel any pain whatsoever. In any event, these men were as impassive as the martyrs whose effigies adorned the entrances of the sanctuaries of relics in the iconography of the twelfth and thirteenth centuries – St Sebastian and St Denis beheaded but cheerfully holding their heads in their hands without a shudder. It was not because pain was not felt, but because it was simply the object of scorn. Pain was not confessed, except by sinners burdened by the excess of their self-criticism and guilt.

However, it seems that this indifference to pain did not last. This restraint in the face of physical pain, this kind of stoicism which repressed any manifestation of emotion when one was confronted with one's own suffering or with the suffering of others, began to end by the late twelfth century. One could ask whether this perceived change expressed in the documents, which give us a glimpse into these feelings, was manifest in the true feelings of the people of that time.

From that time onwards, the sources of information are not limited to those of the Church aristocracy; laymen also begin to express their views. It is at this time, during the fourteenth and fifteenth centuries, that the long process of 'declericalisation' and popularisation of culture begins to reveal progressively the behaviour not only of the heroes of devotion and chivalry, but also of the people. However, it is undeniable that sensitivity, the way of expressing one's passions, did in fact change at all levels of society. This essentially happened as a result of the development of religious consciousness. During the feudal era, a time of great enthusiasm for a pilgrimage to Jerusalem, piety had a tendency to put more emphasis on Jesus himself, to live through a more assiduous meditation on the human nature of the son of God, on his incarnation, and thus on his body and on the fact that the body of Jesus itself experienced pain. Christ was a redeemer because of the immeasurable pain he endured. This pain was immeasurable because it was commensurate with his divinity. This interpretation of the gospel and all the spiritual exercises which accompanied it, the increasing, effective and wide dissemination of these attitudes by such mass media, supported by the artifices of theatre, as were the sermons of the great preachers, gave rise to the progressive valorisation of pain in European

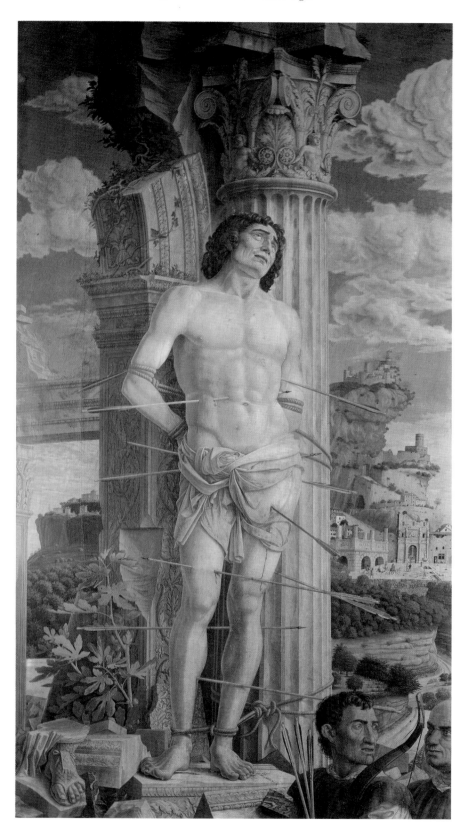

Mantegna *(1431–1506). St. Sebastian.*
(Paris, Musée du Louvre)
(Cl. Giraudon)

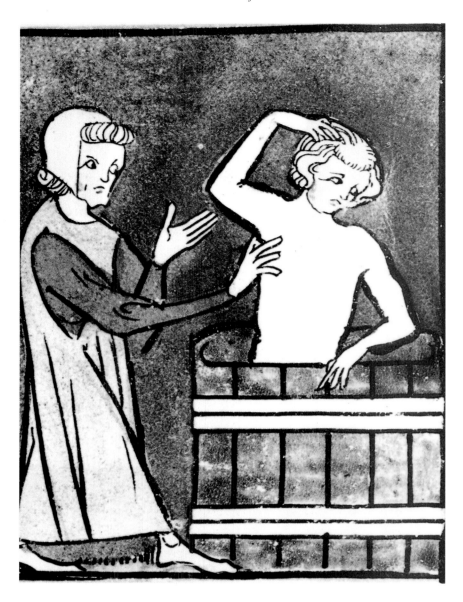

Surgery in the Middle Ages. Practica Rogerii. (British Library MS) (London, Wellcome Institute Library)

culture. Christians were invited to keep in mind the scenes of Passion and physically to place themselves amongst the onlookers of this great spectacle of collective affliction. They were encouraged to imitate Jesus Christ, to identify with the saviour and especially with his physical suffering. There were two milestones in the course of this evolution. To begin with, in the first quarter of the thirteenth century, Francis of Assisi received the stigmata at the height of the expansion of this new devotion. Then, in the first quarter of the fifteenth century, the sudden spread of two pictures were offered for the contemplation of the faithful: the picture of the Man of Pain and that of the Pietá. From then onwards, pain was deliberately brought to the fore. And the emphasis placed upon the suffering body of Jesus was naturally carried over to other suffering bodies such as those of the poor who were the representatives of Christ amongst people on earth. Hence, one can clearly see through the establishment and organisation of charitable institutions and hospitals since the end of the twelfth century, the emergence and development of compassion for the sick, parallel to the development of a piety which sympathises with the pain of flogging and crucifixion. It was as a result of this slow conversion with regard to attitudes towards pain, that medical practice began, although very slowly, to concern itself not only with preparing individuals to learn to die in faith, not only with healing, but also with eliminating the idea that pain as a redeeming punishment was useful to salvation and had to be repressed at all costs, by all means.

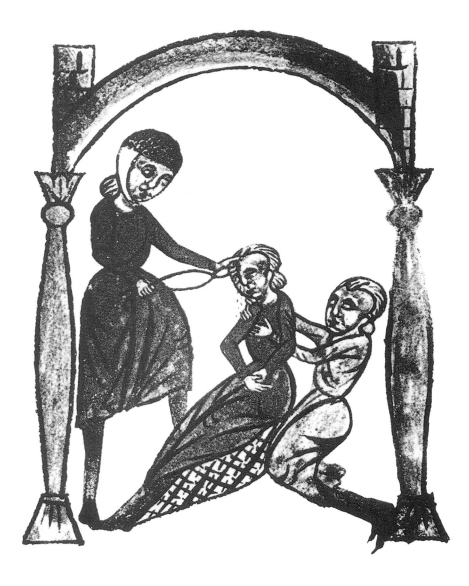

Surgery in the Middle Ages. A female surgeon practising the extraction of an arrow from a patient's head. (Cirurgia Magistri Rolandi, Rome, Biblioteca Casanatense) (London, Wellcome Institute Library)

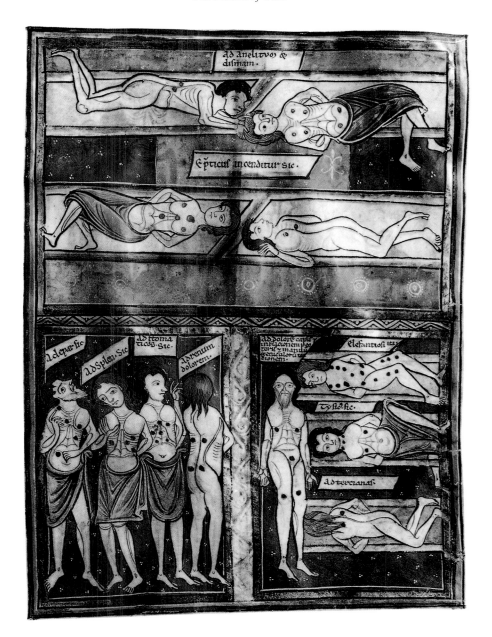

*Points of Cauterisation. Prescribed for
Different Ailments, circa 1200 AD
(Libri Quattuor Medicinae, London,
British Library) (London, Wellcome
Institute Library)*

A Woman in Tears

Marc Le Bot

A WOMAN in tears is one of the symbolic illustrations in Greek mythology that helps us understand the origin of art. This woman is Niobe, Queen of Thebes. She mourns her dead children. The story of this first suffering mother whose face has been painted by artists time and again obeys the same forces that control artistic thought. In both instances, one finds the same faith in the creative production, the same challenge to the divine powers, the same confrontation of pain.

The queen's maternal pride, because she is the fertile mother of seven daughters and seven sons, makes her utter words considered insulting to the power of the gods. So the gods take their revenge. Apollo kills her sons and Artemis her daughters. For nine days and nights, Niobe weeps on their grave. Then she is forced to flee and runs to the top of the frozen heights of Mount Sipyle where Zeus, taking pity on her fate, changes her into a statue of stone. Since then, the waters from heaven have been streaming down her face like the inexhaustible tears of inconsolable pain.

Thus, one of the first statues, one of the first human effigies, is believed to have been the result of the joint work of mourning and a sculptor god, of human pain and the divine sense of the creative artist. So much so that in the arts as well as in the story of Niobe, one finds two similar passions at work: creative arrogance and the confrontation of pain.

In *Antigone*, Sophocles links stone sculpture to pain and death when he describes Niobe: 'Like tenacious ivy, a vegetation of stone imprisons her. All withered, as the story goes, she is continuously covered with rain and snow. And she wets her sides with the tears that eternally flow from her eyelids'.

Here, the stone gradually overcomes the body of Niobe like cold stiffening a dead body. This is because, when it is untreated, lifeless and shapeless, stone is matter; and it is therefore symbolically associated, in the Greek tradition, with death, which is itself motionless, deaf, blind and silent. However, the

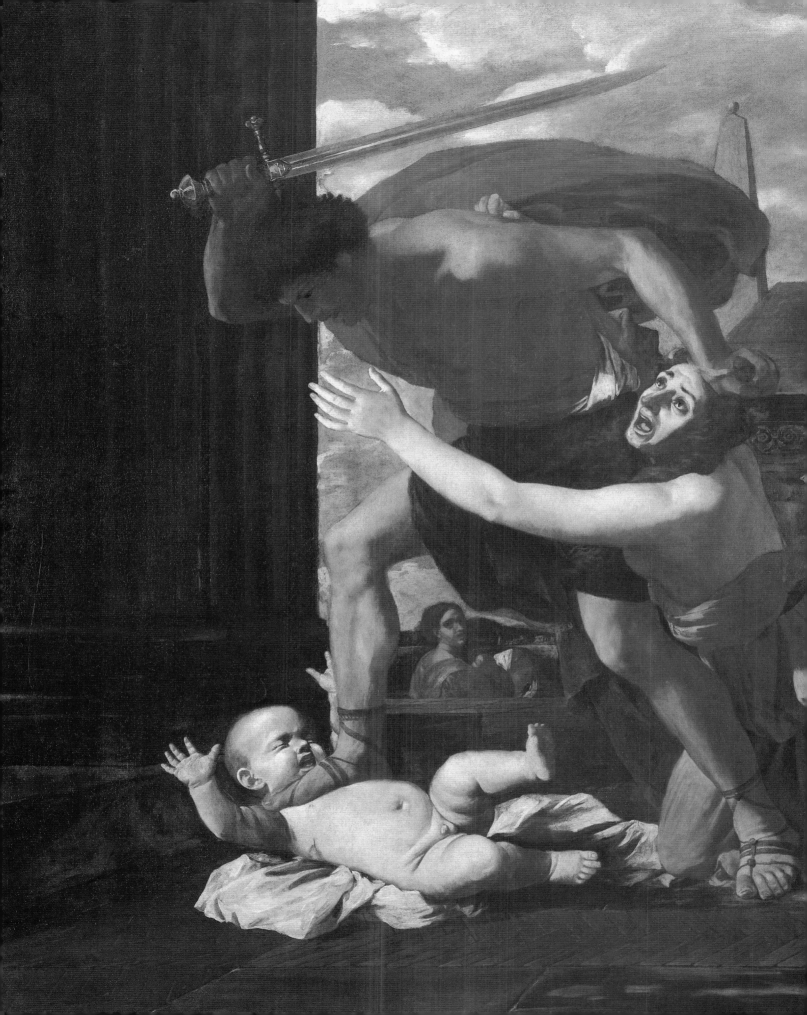

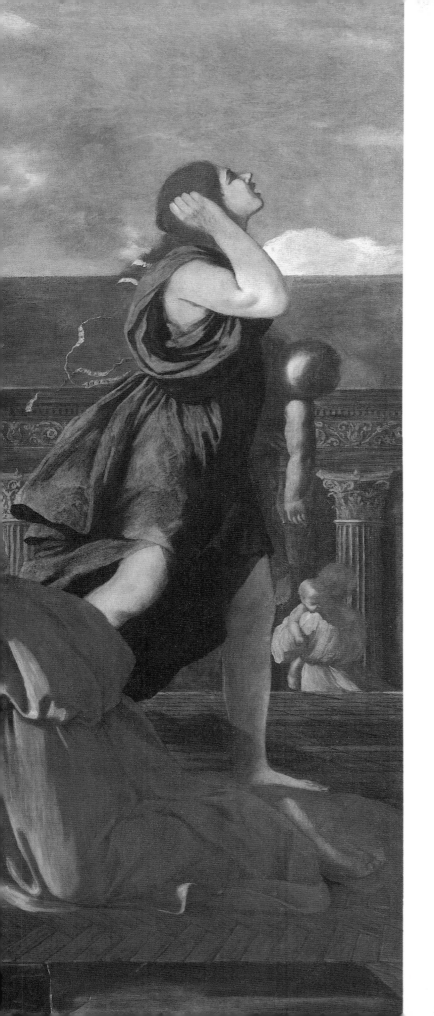

Nicolas Poussin (1594–1665).
The Massacre of the Innocents.
(Chantilly, Condé Museum)
(Giraudon)

same pain that can kill is also the one that, for human beings, creates the vivid representation of their body. And if the nymph Echo is petrified with mourning and becomes a resounding stone that reverberates with the echo of human cries, the art of the sculptor is also, conversely, the one that gives life to matter, as when Galatea comes to life under the chisel of Pygmalion.

This was the perception of art in Greece. The painted or sculptured images arrest the movement of the living individual; they freeze it in a motionless representation equivalent to a symbolic death. Nevertheless, the presence of these replicas before our eyes breathes a second life into the missing ones and into the dead. Art is at the frontier where life and death face each other. And the Greeks might have conceived that one of art's origins lay in the encounter between humans and pain.

More recently, Francis Bacon took up the same idea linking the representation of the human body with inconsolable grief and the image of the woman in tears. However, he refuses to accept that his works are 'illustrations' of some story or other. According to Bacon, art is only for the sake of art; it has no story to tell. But, symbolically, he put the idea test through a mixture of life and

Giotto (1266–1337).
Lamentation on the dead Christ.
(Padoue, Chapelle des Scrovegni)
(Giraudon)

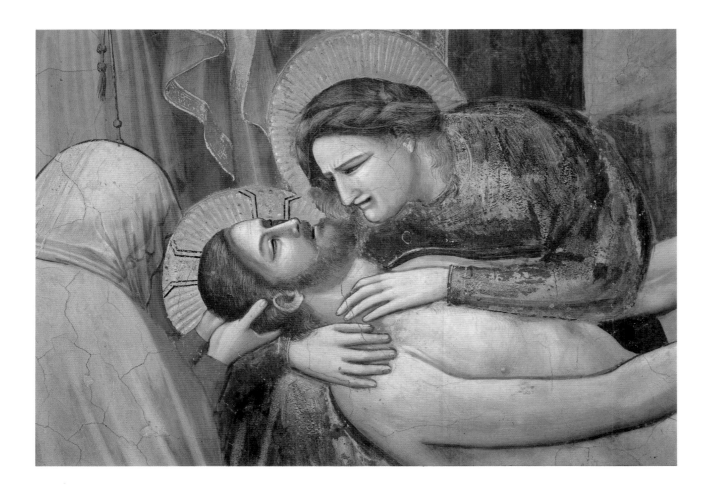

death, love and hate, happiness and pain. He says, in essence: 'I was hoping one day to paint the best picture of the human cry. I have not been able to do so … I believe that the best painting of the cry was made by Poussin.'

In *The Massacre of the Innocents*, by Nicolas Poussin in the 1630s, the woman who cries with her mouth wide open is kneeling down and her body bends forward. Her posture reminds us of a long tradition of women in pain in the art of painting. The first, no doubt, are the holy women lamenting the death of Christ, painted by Giotto at Padoue, *circa* 1320. Here, for the first time, the picture of the human body is rescued from the fixedness of stereotypes. It becomes quite important, quite expressive. Giotto suggests that individuals achieve their own destiny through action; but this action is also where they come face to face with pain.

A century later, in the Carmine Church at Florence, Masaccio has the intuition that there is something very deep about pain for the modern man and woman. According to him, the gap between the two is the result of an original loss beyond repair. And pain therefore is not one of those dead and hard stones that one stumbles over. For Masaccio, pain is an origin: an intense source of our thoughts. Here, for the first time, pain is totally human.

This is because, in Giotto's paintings, the space within which men and women act is limited by the scenery of the stage; and this fixed space gives the representation of women in tears, like that of Niobe, something of the stiffness of stone statues. On the contrary, the space that encloses the figures in Masaccio's work is akin to an abyss. These images are caught in an interplay of shadows, lights and colours that opens the space into an inaccessible infinity. Masaccio links this idea of infinitude with that of pain. Adam and Eve, as he paints them, no longer show signs of the stiffness of the statues. Light and colours frame their bodies in a space that welcomes them; and yet, one's eyes reach into infinity.

And because one is looking at a vanishing horizon, God and His paradise are from now on the ones missing from the terrestrial scenes; they are the irreparable loss of our vision into infinity. The bottomless space becomes the concrete image of painful anguish as the painter reveals that it is this anguish that sets the bodies into motion. Hence, Adam's right leg is bent into a curve as though he refuses to pull it away from the ground of the Garden of Eden; his face in tears which he hides in his hands signifies our pain. And 'the most beautiful human cry' – Eve's black and wide open mouth – is no doubt also the first to have been painted.

Francis Bacon also painted crying men. In Bacon's work, the representations of pain are connected with pondering the powers and weaknesses of men, over an abyss that opens up under their feet at the very moment they reach the pinnacle of power and glory.

When painting the crying man, Bacon draws inspiration from the effigy of Pope Innocent X, painted by Velasquez in 1650 in Rome. Bacon says of the Spanish painter that he seems in this instance 'to go for a walk on the brink of

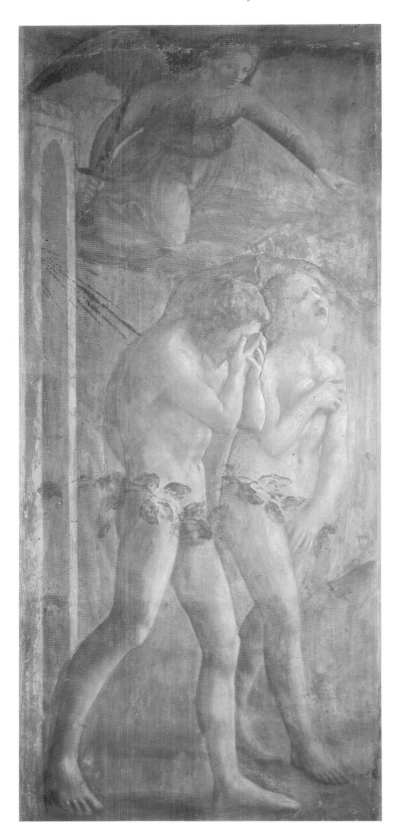

Tommaso Masaccio *(1401–1428).*
Adam and Eve driven out of Paradise.
(Basilica del Carmine, Florence)
(Bridgeman Art Library)

the precipice – to open up entirely to the biggest and most profound things that a man can feel'. In his own paintings, the symbol of these profound things, the precipice or abyss, is also a black mouth that is wide open. But mainly, following the example of Velasquez, Bacon is working on making signs of violence and pain part of the art of painting.

In Velasquez's effigy of Innocent X, the folds of the red curtains form a space as solemn as that of a temple or palace; the seat of the pontiff as well as its rectangular frame bear testimony to the same solemnity of power that marks the features of the face. However, the surplice of the pope is a smear of white streaks, as if, suddenly, the visible was smashed into pieces. A similar tension between shape, shapelessness and intense colours is also found in Bacon's work, between large monochromatic flat tints and pictures that are overcome by violence; but a geometric structure, similar to the one formed by the seat of Innocent X, prevents them from falling back into magma. At this point the images in the painting cry out and their mouths open wide onto a black abyss.

In Bacon's *Crucifixions*, the sorrowful figures (those perhaps of Magdalene and Mary standing around the cross, or of the Greek Furies, as the painter points out) are bodies distorted by pain to the point of becoming monsters.

So, we men and women are driven by a force that teaches us our place and destroys us at the same time. The enigma of the human condition is the duality that the artist is confronted with when dealing with opposites. Life and death are inseparable; pain is the nadir of human glory; love and hate are head and tail of the same coin. These ambivalences stir up a feeling of terror in us and our thoughts confront this terror through pain.

Francis Bacon, in what he calls the 'reality' of human beings and things, is in fact undergoing a strange and difficult experience. He denies that it is the love versus hate dichotomy. And he also denies that it is disturbing or that it generates fear. He talks about it in terms of vertigo and abyss.

Bacon in fact maintains he only paints portraits of friends, and only from photographs, in their absence. 'I would be inhibited' he says, 'if I had to carry out the attack I inflict on them in my work in their presence. I prefer to carry out in private the attack through which I feel I can record their reality more accurately.'

But he is categorical: no affective ambivalence is in question here. Art does not have to get into 'psychological judgements': 'It reaches down to something more profound: How is it that I feel that I can make this picture much more real for me? That's all … What I want to achieve is a distortion of the object and a separation between it and its representation, and out of this distortion a restoration of the object to a recording of the representation involved.'

He asks, 'Who, nowadays, has been able to record anything and has succeeded in making it affect the world as a reality without making a profound attack on the picture?' That is because 'nowadays' we are 'outside tradition'. We are unprotected. We lack the myths and the legends that, not so long ago, allowed art to reflect upon the human condition. All we can do now is in fact 'record' what is. We are naked before the naked reality of the others, before their surprising otherness. And we are driven, in comparison to them, by intense feelings that we can tell have the power of crushing everything in their path. So much so that, in confronting them, we experience a feeling of fear.

In trying to understand how, in the work of Francis Bacon, these crushing forces are applied to the human image and are still restrained by the lines and colours in flat tints, one realises that art endeavours to translate the love–hate dichotomy and the anguish or the fear that is always the result of this ambivalence, into an experience of a breathtaking abyss. This experience clearly precedes or goes beyond common psychological reactions. Art reaches down for the 'most profound', it reaches deep down for what is in the heart. Velasquez sees and invites others to see Pope Innocent X in his strength, a strength that is also his weakness. Francis Bacon, in his *Crucifixions*, is fascinated because the 'high and isolated' position of Christ is also a position occupied by a dead man.

Art is therefore, according to Bacon, a form of thought that faces up to, and forces us to face up to, the astounding experience of the enormous gap, and yet an identity that separates and unites 'the greatness and downfall': love and hate, life and death. Velasquez faces up to it with 'miraculous' sovereignty. Like him, 'one would like … to do this thing which simply consists of going for a walk on the brink of the precipice'. One would like art to be a form of thought whereby one faces up to one's own destiny by overcoming one's fears.

Francis Bacon probably succeeds in doing this. He finds in art a chance to keep his fears at arm's length. At least he strove to do so: 'You could say that a cry is a picture of horror; in fact, it is the cry more than the horror that I wanted to paint … I like everything that shines and the colour that comes from the mouth, and I was hoping … to be able to paint the mouth like Monet painted the sunset.'

According to Giacometti, the experience of life and death and the terrible fear that ensues is at the heart of artistic work. This experience is that of the other, who is both present and absent for us and at once infinitely close and distant. A disturbing strangeness is obvious as soon as we cast a naive or naked look at the others, ignorant of their knowledge and habits and charged only with passionate attention.

Then, writes Giacometti observing a face, suddenly 'the shape becomes undone, it is no more than particles in motion on a black and deep emptiness, the distance between one nostril and the other is like the Sahara; there are no frontiers, nothing to gaze at, everything escapes …'

'I began to see heads in the emptiness, in the space that surrounds them. When, for the first time, I saw the head I was looking at become still, suddenly and definitively fixed into position, I trembled with terror as I never did before and I could feel a cold sweat running down my back. It was no longer a living head, but an object I was looking at, like any other object; no, not like any other object, but rather like something that was both alive and dead at the same time. I shouted out in terror, as if I had just crossed a threshold, as though I was

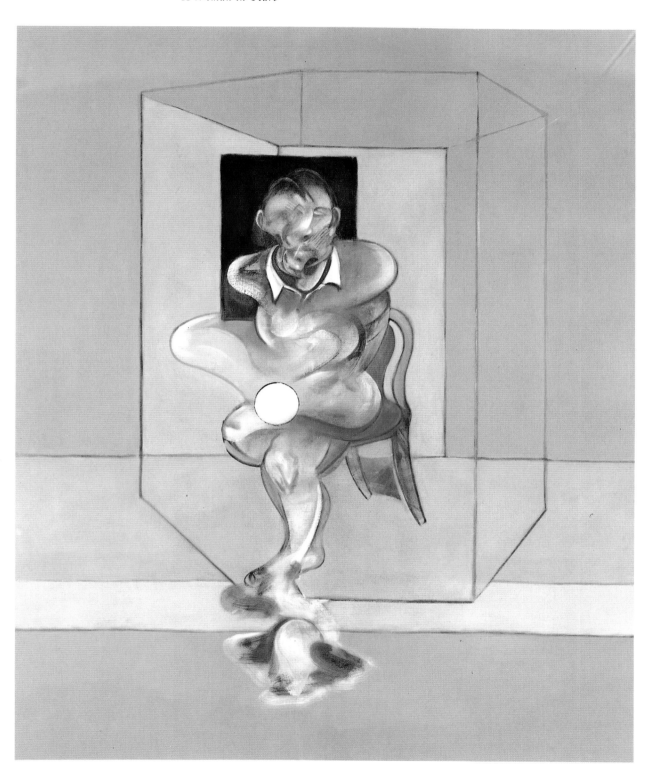

Francis Bacon *(1909–1992).*
Study for a Self-portrait.
(Claude Bernard Gallery)

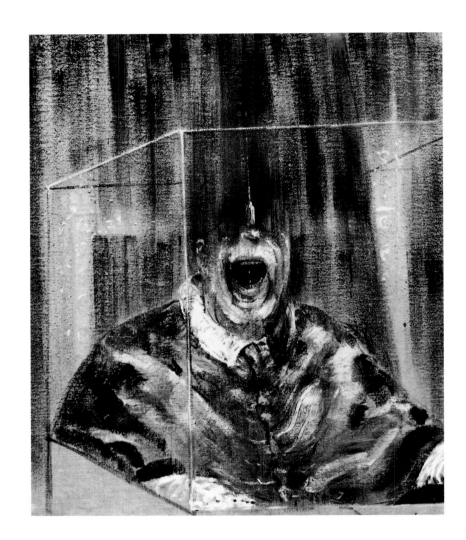

Francis Bacon *(1909–1992).*
Head VI 1949.
(Arts Council Collection)
(Claude Bernard Gallery)

opposite page:
Francis Bacon *(1909–1992).*
Three Studies for the Human Body.
(Claude Bernard Gallery)

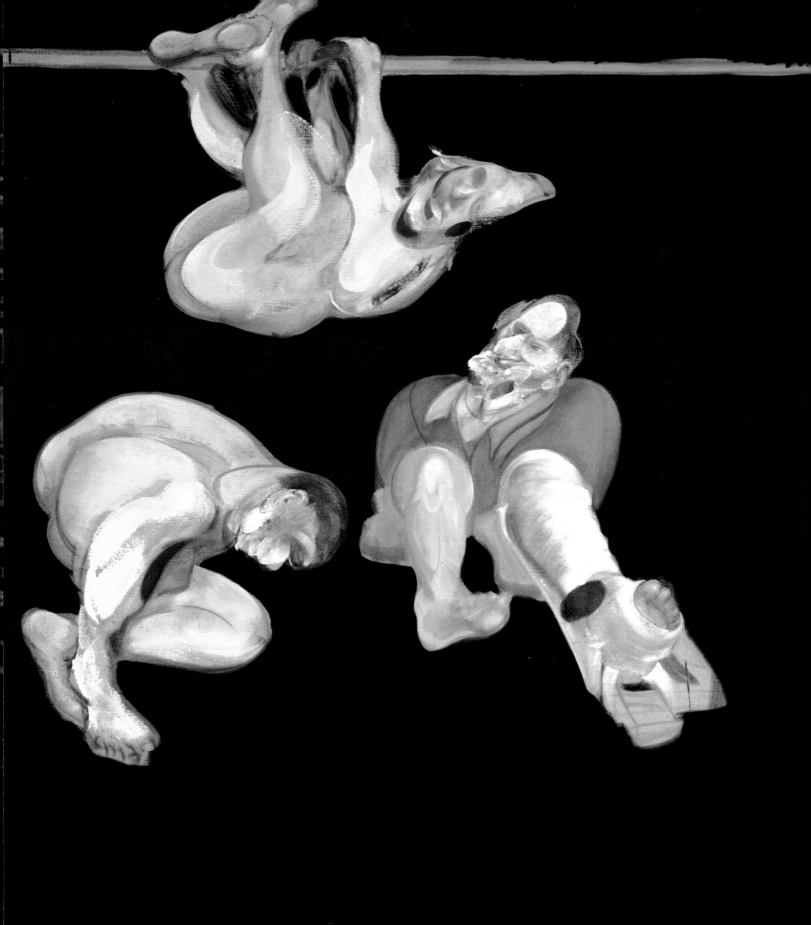

entering a new world. All the living were dead ...'

Panic or fear is accompanied by mortal pain in the work of Vladimir Velick-ovic. Male nudes desperately try to run away; they leap in spaces that are closed and are closing in on them, their tints often reduced to black and white. Other images are in the hereafter of pain. There are bodies hanging from hooks and ropes, victims of dismemberment or torture, or bodies stretched out on a tombstone. The suffering causes spasms in the bodies; the muscles and bones twitch. Yet this suffering touches us in more profound ways: it takes root in the substance of the painting and through visual effects assails our eyes.

Velickovic's paintings convey all the cruelty and fear that is possible. They exert a fascination over us. There is no painting, even one of a happy scene, that does not end by arousing in us a feeling of strangeness and anxiety. This is because our minds, no matter how hard we try, can never get a sure hold on the painting. Something visible is there but it is always a double vision. It is what we see as well as the impression of movements by the artist's hand. In front of any painting, we know that nothing we can say will explain the strangeness of this dual presence.

Velickovic pushes this anxiety to its extremes, to representation of violence and pain. His paintings petrify us. His images remind us of the Gorgon herself: the eyes of Medusa killed those who looked upon her, transforming victims into blocks of stone. Velickovic has often painted bodies running away or eager to run away; but the pictorial effects seem to freeze them in space. In his paintings people panic and suffer. But it is only an effect of the painting. Velickovic's nudes are painted with a full brush, muscle after muscle, with crushed faces and blood everywhere. They form a whirlwind of vivid colours, but the tormented bodies are often depicted in neutral and almost black tints painted flat. Thus the terrible opposition between painful spasms and a fixed space is played out before our eyes.

These effects mesmerise. The viewer is truly petrified. But recent paintings by Velickovic develop the concept of motionless time. In a slow, very slow way, they return to motion. The large monochromatic flat tints that formed the background of his paintings are substituted with what the painter calls 'landscapes'. A few shapes indicate open areas where there is nothing else but walls and enclosures: a road, a bare tree trunk with a branch, sometimes a dog that goes round in a circle. However, large areas of flat colours remain. Two different spaces and two different times seem to coexist in these paintings: the motionlessness remains, whereas the mechanism of a spectacle finds in it a temporal and spatial rhythm.

Paradoxically, this tension between frozen time and time that appears to be in motion makes both times coexist. One questions the true nature of tragic space and time. Space and time take charge and pain is sublimated. Tragedy directs and initiates destinies which have been in play since eternity. What people of antiquity called Destiny is what is at stake in a time of paradox: our lives make happen what was supposed to happen in any event and this some-

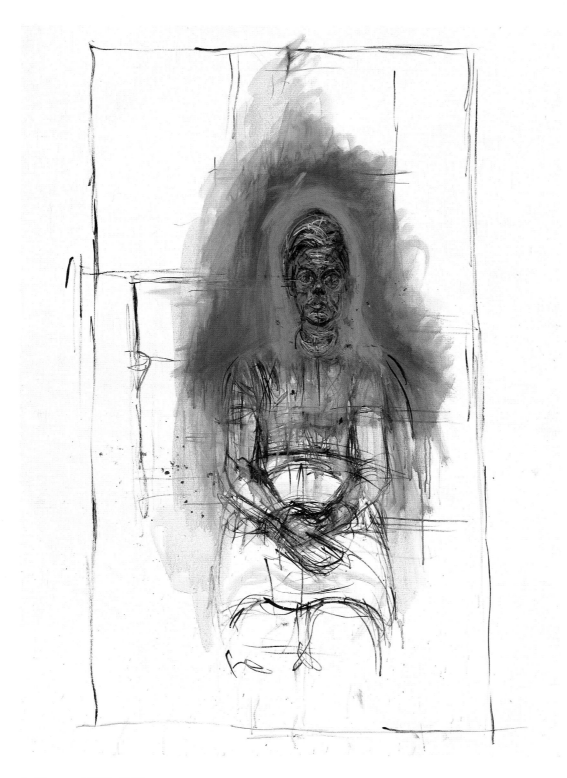

A. Giacometti *(1901–1966).*
Caroline. (Georges Pompidou Centre)

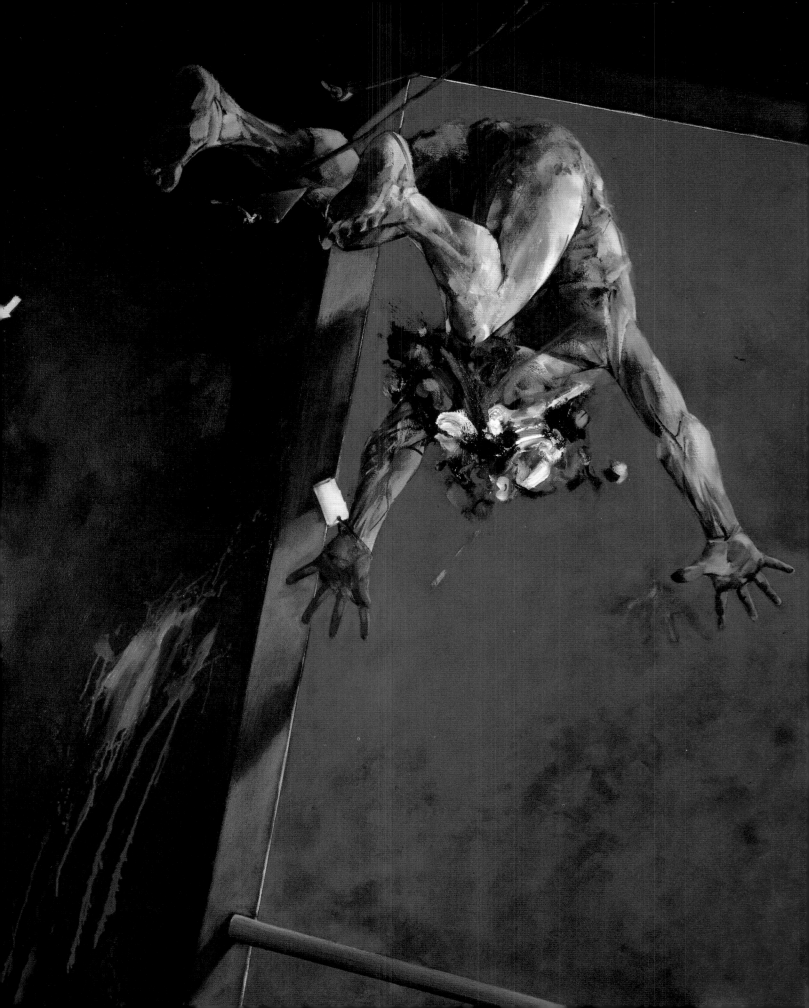

how takes us by surprise. Something in destiny is unintelligible to us: at both ends of time blood flows. We are born to life from nothingness and return to this same nothingness in death.

Violence and cruelty, representations of bloody births and deaths, of scorched and tortured bodies, take on an allegorical value in this kind of painting; we confront human time with pain but also with a passion for life.

Some painters, and such examples are very rare, tell us to confront what causes us the most obscure fears, what Rainer Maria Rilke calls 'the terrifying'. Their paintings ask: what is left of the human when we happen to venture within the limits of the inhuman? Quite a number of paintings by Jean Rustin are terrifying. The figures in these paintings have their eyes open on something that cannot be contemplated without trembling with fear. Yet the eyes are transfixed in peaceful meditation. These paintings are based on the same feeling of piety and pity that once made artists paint pietàs and crucifixions.

The paintings of Jean Rustin refer to that which is most terrifying: the double defeat of the body and the spirit, decrepitude and idiocy. The images of these paintings proffer pain, a dull but sometimes violent pain as we have all experienced during hard times. Its obviousness overwhelms us and captures our attention before we can identify the images of the human bodies. There is visual confusion caused by the haze of ochres. The coloured matter vibrates because of the painstaking technique of tints applied patiently by a repetitive hand. Here, light moves from darkness back to light and vice versa, through imperceptible degrees, and the colours join in a common vibration that intensifies their vividness. The result is very much like the effect of encircling. All that is visible – the human representations, the places and things – seem to have been made out of unique matter, to have been carved in one block of motionless space. We find ourselves caught up in this, and threatened by anxiety caused by bewildered immobility. The conquered and distorted bodies are left to the forces of destruction, but we know that these forces commit acts of violence on our spirits and bodies, before they defeat and kill us.

This violence and its accompanying anxiety are feelings we find very hard to rationalise. In our Christian tradition, the strongest symbolic representation is that of the Virgin mourning her dead son, first at the cross, then at his grave. Like the representation of Niobe in the Greek legend, the Pietà shows the extreme pain of the Christian tradition. It is this maternal pain that distorts the shape of the monster-like figures that Francis Bacon painted in his *Crucifixions*. And it is the Pietà that Jean Rustin reminded us of when, in 1982, he painted *Image Pieuse (A Pious Image)*.

There are two women in this painting. Both are nude and both are dead. And death itself is already present. Together, they are on a threshold, like the mother of Christ holding her dead son in her arms next to his grave. In the Pietà, as in this insane image, two bodies watch over these two women on the brink of the absolute limit where everything is obstructed: nothing ever becomes what it might have been because it comes upon madness and death.

opposite page:
Vladimir Velickovic.
Exit. (Frac Alsace Collection)

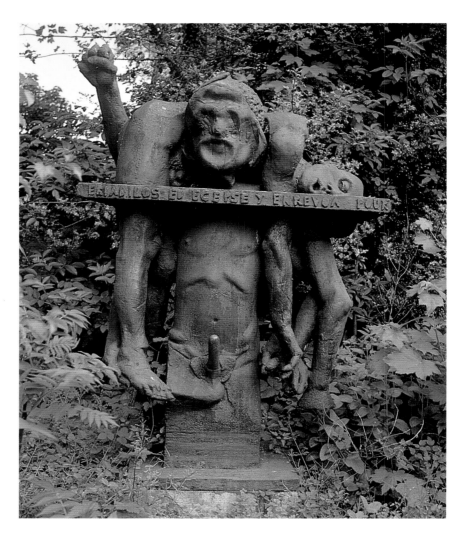

Ipousteguy
The death of the brother.

The boundary is not to be crossed. It is everywhere. A deserted land has opened up. That is why there are two women, just like the mother and her dead son. The emptiness is the common place where every self meets their own other self. In other words, this space of nothingness, where everyone loses oneself, is internal. Madness and death separate me from my ego. Each dead body is separated from its body. The spirit bumps into something as the head bumps against the wall. How is it possible that these women are not mad? The same madness is reflected in the blindness of the eyes, every time they avoid the unbearable image. He who runs away from the image of these distorted bodies on the verge of the abyss of nothingness, also runs away from the double of his own body, when something within him offers itself to defeat.

A painting is unbearable when it carries within it the death of meaning itself. But is there a painting that does not carry this death of meaning? Art, if we are to capture all of its effects, cannot fail to evoke a dangerous anxiety in us. Art makes things visible to us; but it also makes this visibility full of devices that conceal the very meaning of art. The enigma of the visible, with its inherent nonsense, madness and death, is the end result of the act of seeing.

Then nothing. Only naked visibility remains. It is there like raw material. And yet, art gives to this a sensitive skin, as sensitive as the skin of a body. The aim of art is therefore to convey to us the painful strangeness of familiar things. It rekindles our fears in order to control them.

Pain and History in the Western World

Roy Porter

Contradictions of the Western World

PAIN is one of the great enigmas of Western history. Attitudes towards it have been profoundly contradictory, and theory and practice have been deeply at odds. Pain has commonly been regarded as a consummate evil, and freedom from pain has often been represented as a great goal of human life, as exemplified by the elevated 'apathy' of the Stoic philosopher or the peace of the Christian heaven. Yet governments and ideologies have frequently seemed hellbent upon the calculated intensification of pain and suffering. Alongside the inevitable agonies of pestilence and famine and the uncontrollable carnage of the battlefield, political regimes have traditionally gone in for the deliberate, formal, and systematic infliction of pain, well beyond obvious rational necessity. Take for instance the public execution, universal in European states until at least the close of the eighteenth century: a symbolic act of ferocity which we may view as the state-authorised pursuit of cruelty.

A Wrong for a Right

From Naples to Hamburg, the public execution as the enactment of the 'triumph of justice' was staged as an exemplary civic pageant. Fettered and scourged, the condemned person might be dragged behind a horse on a long parade through the streets to the place of execution, where tortures would be inflicted – the whip or rack, strappado or wheel – followed by what was often an extremely protracted death, by hanging, crucifixion, or burning alive; stoning to death was not an officially sanctioned mode of justice in Europe, though it doubtlessly occurred. The expiring or dead body was then commonly quartered, dismembered, and defiled. Well-documented cases like that of Damiens, the would-be assassin of Louis XV, show that the procedures of judicial execution might last several days, and even then a severed head might be spiked and the corpse left to hang in chains until it rotted, to frighten children and the poor. This entire spectacle was meant to excite maximum public horror. For instance, this execution scene, was recalled by the Swiss doctor, Felix Platter, in the sixteenth century:

'A criminal, having raped a seventy-year old woman, was flayed alive with burning tongs. With mine own eyes, I saw the thick smoke produced by his living flesh that had been subjected to the tongs. The prisoner was a strong, vigorous man. On the bridge over the Rhine, just nearby, they tore out his breast; then he was led to the scaffold. By now he was extremely feeble and blood was gushing from his hands. He could no longer remain standing; he fell down continually. Finally he was decapitated. They drove a stake through his body, and then his corpse was thrown into a ditch. I myself was witness to his torture, my father holding me by the hand.'

As was common in those times, the child had been taken to watch the execution by his father, to teach him a moral lesson.

To anyone who might innocently think that capital punishment was a simple act of retribution (an eye for an eye), a technique of penalising crime and deterring criminals, the sheer superabundance of cruelty involved in such public tortures and executions must appear gratuitous and grotesque. Indeed, that was precisely what reformers – particularly the *philosophes* of the Enlightenment – were to argue. Nevertheless there were plenty of defenders of the

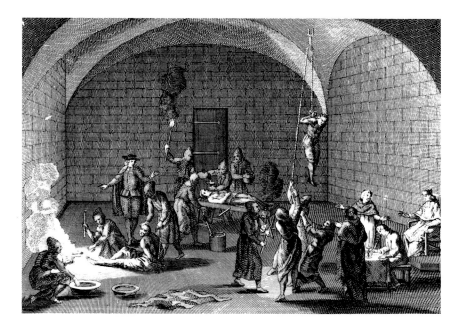

B. Picart *(1737). Torture chamber during the Inquisition.*
(Mary Evans Picture Library)

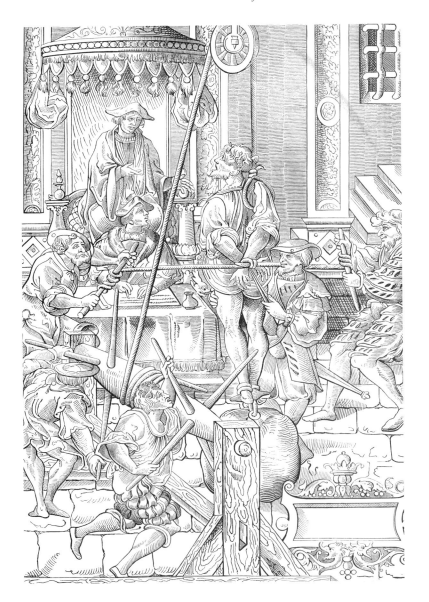

The Strappado, 'Extraordinary Question'.
Facsimile of a painting on wood by
J. Millaeus. Praxis Criminis Persequendi,
Paris, 1541.
(Mary Evans Picture Library)

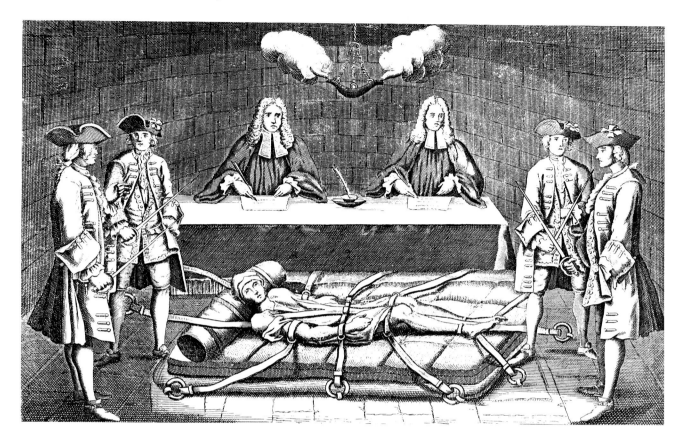

*The Torture of Damiens, before his attempt
to assassinate Louis XV, 1757.
(Mary Evans Picture Library)*

administration of 'surplus pain'. Apologists argued that the excruciating intensity of death agonies would extract full confessions of truth, public declarations of guilt and contrition, a humbling of the culprit, and perhaps an ultimate religious conversion. If the death throes were sufficiently extreme, the criminal on his *via crucis* might even be enabled, thanks to the severity of the pain, finally to die 'a good death'. There were, by all accounts, instances in which tortured offenders did indeed pray fervently and lead the assembled throngs in fervent ejaculations. Yet, in engraving after engraving, William Hogarth shows us the reverse side of this public theatre of cruelty: the drunken crowds at Tyburn jeering and joshing the blaspheming, impenitent convict. Partly because violence so obviously bred violence, in the end the reformers had their way. The administration of capital punishment became 'humane' and private, before it was, in civilised nations, finally abolished. But the question remains: what explains this apparent dedication to the systematic perpetration of unnecessary pain?

The public execution was not unique. In many other respects, the infliction of pain was part of the official fabric of traditional society. Criminal statutes,

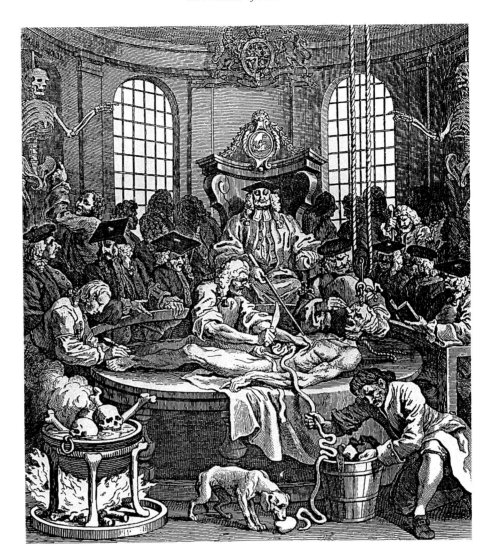

William Hogarth *(1697–1764). Punishment*
for Cruelty. Anonymous engraving after Hogarth,
1751. (London, Wellcome Institute Library)

torturers' manuals, penal systems, religious exercises: all encode a culture of
pain. And that is to say nothing of the taste for sadomasochism, which was
evidently deeply rooted long before it achieved visibility in the writings of the
Marquis de Sade (1740–1814). A long reflective tradition in art and literature
pointed out the pleasures of melancholy, the pained heart.

All such forms of authorised pain are worth pondering, because they exem-
plify the immensely perplexing attitudes towards pain embedded in the
philosophies of law, public enactments and opinion. Pain is simultaneously
viewed as an evil in itself, yet also, potentially, the most powerful instrument
for bringing about good.

A Taboo Subject

There is a second way in which pain is difficult to grasp historically. Understanding pain must be central to understanding politics and power, yet it has also typically eluded discussion. Relatively few of the great works of our culture – religious, philosophical, ethical – have made *pain* their fundamental focus. Philosophy has been more concerned with establishing the nature of virtue, theology with the salvation of the soul. It is even arguable that medicine itself customarily put pain control and relief fairly low on its list of priorities.

It is remarkable how late anaesthetics were developed – not until the 1840s – or how recently the pharmaceutical industry began to devote itself to developing improved analgesics. Even psychiatry was slow to focus attention on pain; in itself, it was not a topic central to Freud's lifelong investigations. It is said that the understanding of pain formed no direct part of psychiatric training before the 1960s. In a sense, pain, though omnipresent – perhaps *because* it was ubiquitous – was hardly to be talked about.

Several reasons for this can be suggested. Pain suffers guilt-by-association because of its proximity to matters physical and carnal. Powerful cultural traditions, especially evident in the Anglo-Saxon world, have made the body a taboo topic. The body is inferior to the mind or spirit; it is inherently dirty and degrading. It is a symptom of weakness or prurience to pay too much

William Hogarth (1697–1764). The lazy apprentice is put to death at Tyburn. Engraving by T. Cook, after Hogarth. (London, Wellcome Institute Library)

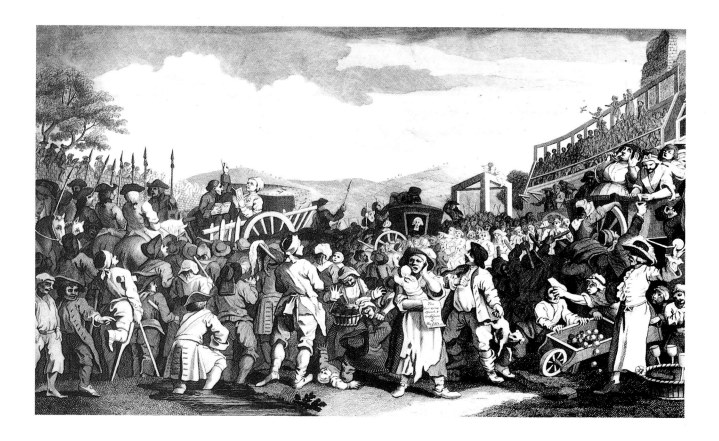

attention to its wants, needs and demands – people are expected to be more 'high minded'. The same has obviously been true in the shaping of outlooks on pain. Notably in the Victorian era, agonies were to be endured with a stiff upper lip. This was doubtless good practical advice, especially in centuries where effective pharmaceutical agents of pain control were scarcely available. But it was also symptomatic of a wider, elitist contempt for the flesh and its afflictions.

This disparagement of the senses is, of course, highly apparent in the ways in which Western society, especially during the last two or three centuries, has categorised different sorts of pain and the bodily defects and diseases pain supposedly indicates. Powerful traditions within medicine have been keen to adjudge pain as 'real' only when it can be related to obvious physical causes: a tumour, inflammation or a wound. 'Real pain, especially severe pain', argued the distinguished US physician, Walter Alvarez (1884-1978), 'points to the presence of organic rather than functional disease.' The professional appeal of such a view is obvious. It grounds pain in biomedicine, makes it subject to the laws of nature, takes the mystery out of pain, and thereby gives promise for its cure. Alvarez continued as follows: 'On the other hand, a burning, or a quivering, or a picking, pricking, pulling, pumping, crawling, boiling, gurgling, thumping, throbbing, gassy or itching sensation, or a constant ache, or soreness, strongly suggests a neurosis.'

Alvarez's discomfort with the protean nature of pain was obvious. He was clearly aware that there were pains that were difficult to pin down to any palpable organ in the body. Therefore he felt the need to confront the possibility, either that they were feigned – the work of a malingerer – or that they were tricks played by the unconscious upon psychologically maladjusted or highly suggestible individuals.

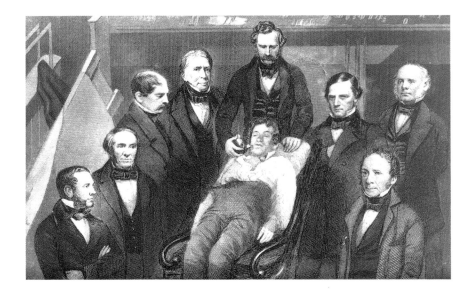

W.T.G. Morton carrying out an etherisation in public for the first time at the Massachusetts General Hospital. Painting by H.B. Hall. (London, Wellcome Institute Library)

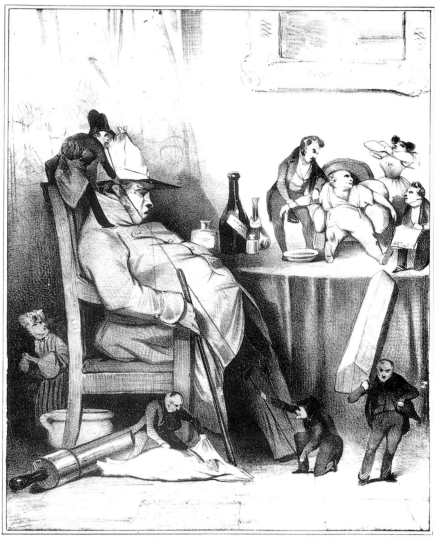

Le malade imaginaire.

Je suis perdu il faut faire mon testament ils vont m'ensevelir m'encore adieu

The Imaginary Invalid.
A hypochondriac thinking about the
preparations for his burial.
(London, Wellcome Institute Library)

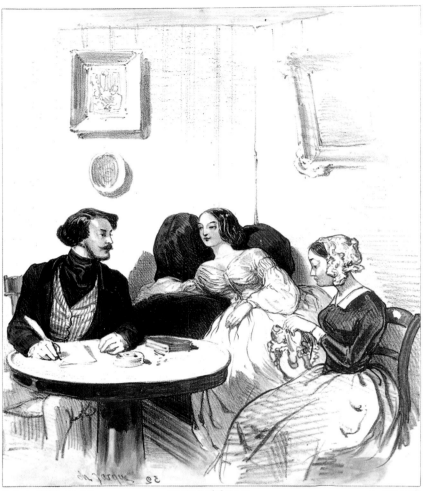

LE MÉDECIN DE DAMES.

— Pour calmer cette névralgie voici mon ordonnance : Vous prendrez ce soir une loge aux Variétés demain une loge à l'Opéra....et en outre je tâcherai de faire prendre par votre mari ce cachemire vert que vous avez vu chez Gagelin et que vous désirez tant !...

— Ah! docteur, vous êtes un homme charmant !...

Charles-Émile Jacques (1813–1894).
The Ladies' Doctor, a medical practitioner
prescribing recreational activities to a young
woman suffering from a nervous disease.
(London, Wellcome Institute Library)

Painful to Express

These matters lay bare a profound ambivalence in our society to the act of giving expression to pain. Though experienced directly only by the patient, its expression (in screams, words or gestures) seeks psycho-physiological discharge, but also hopes to elicit sympathy; the person who adopts what the US sociologist Talcott Parsons called the 'sick role' expects some secondary gain. But the stereotype of the *malade imaginaire* that achieved notoriety from the eighteenth century – the patient whose disorders were created or exacerbated by a 'warm imagination' – suggests that such a performance was always liable to excite suspicion and resistance amongst a public on its guard against those making a meal, or a career, out of pain.

Too fluent a talent for articulating agonies aroused fears that they were mere rhetoric or histrionics; greater sympathy was often accorded to those who suffered in silence. In our culture it has been permissible to have a 'complaint', but not to be a 'complainer'. Physicians of the Victorian era in particular thought it was dangerous to allow patients to supply overly graphic accounts of their pains, lest this encourage morbid introspection. Faced with patients who dwelt on their troubles, physicians widely advocated diversionary activities, to induce sufferers to forget, and cease talking about, their conditions: riding, sport, fresh air, massage, and the 'rest cure' developed in the US by George Beard (1839–1883) and Silas Weir Mitchell (1829–1914). Sent to a nursing home to recover from her 'nervous breakdown', Virginia Woolf (1882–1941) was denied pen and paper, books and visitors, in the rather naive hope of taking her mind off her troubles. The Anglo-Saxon ideal of pain involved a preferred idiom of understatement. The true Englishman might be doubled up with pain, with one foot in the grave, but was meant to respond to health inquiries with a reassuring 'a bit under the weather' or 'a little off colour'.

All this talk of hypochondria takes for granted that it is valid to draw some distinction between 'real' pain and 'neurotic' pain. This is, at bottom, a question for the neurobiologists. But, from the historical viewpoint, making the distinction is inherently problematic, not to say question-begging. For pain is irreducibly subjective. Whatever it may signal or express, pain is *felt*, is a sensation – or, better, an experience – and thus exists in the mind or psyche.

The rather suspect urge to differentiate between 'physical' and 'mental' pain that we have encountered in Alvarez, of course, has resulted in the creation of the category of what have been called, for the last century, psychosomatic disorders: conditions in which, although the sick person feels the pain associated with organic disease, the medical profession judges that no real ('organic') disease is present. From the standpoint of the suffering patient, it would seem more humane to accept the validity of psychosomatic illnesses, without feeling the need to judge some pains more 'real' than others, with its inevitable consequence of downgrading the experience of those whose pains are deemed 'subjective'.

Pain is thus problematic in the sphere of historical facts because it is an *experience*; it is subjective, and here, more or less, private, and unique to each individual. This has meant that, for centuries, pain has actually proved very difficult to articulate or discuss in a satisfactory, intelligible language. Fleeting and internal, pain is difficult to measure and hard to verbalise, at least with any precision. As has often been remarked, illness tends to reduce even the most articulate to states of mute misery or meaningless noise. Reflecting sympathetically upon the hypochondriac's plight, Thomas Beddoes (1760-1808), the prominent Bristol physician, remarked that 'the hypochondria sufferer always finds language fails him, when he gives vent to his complaints'. Whatever words he uttered inevitably sounded inadequate or anticlimactic: 'He tells you he has heart burn, dreadful flatulence', and so forth, but these were at best distant approximations to his actual sensations. And so, 'after vain and unsatisfactory efforts, his conclusion generally is, 'In short you see before you, the most miserable wretch upon the face of the earth'. Beddoes put his finger on the problem of grasping other people's pain or expressing one's own. Language was perhaps a good tool for representing tangible objects in the natural, external world (a chair, a tree). By contrast, Beddoes contended, 'language has not yet been adjusted with any degree of exactness, to our inward feelings. Hence medical reports, where these feelings come in question, stand a double chance of inaccuracy. The invalid, with whom the representation must originate, may express himself ill (*sic!*); and the physician may misconceive him if he takes him simply at his word, or by trying to help him out, may substitute his own ideas. How little then can we depend upon generalisation of such obscure data!'

Indeed, the very notion of a syntax of pain has been culturally and morally problematic. Over the centuries, it has often been argued that physical outrages or emotional injuries may be so terrible that to translate them into words may obscenely traduce and degrade them; we talk after fall of 'unspeakable' atrocities. Silence may be more eloquent than speech. 'The rest is silence': great playwrights like Shakespeare have recognised that the dramatic presentation of tragedy is readily trivialised by descriptive vocabulary. In the depths of his pain, the words King Lear utters are 'Howl, howl, howl, howl, howl'.

With Nazi extermination-camp tortures in mind, the critic George Steiner has contended that abominations may be so excruciating, physiologically and psychologically, as to be beyond the healing power of words, and even perhaps the redemptive capacity of art. And, in *The Body in Pain*, an exhaustive discussion of the place of pain in the Judaeo-Christian theodicy and in later secular metaphysics, the literary historian, Elace Scarry, has noted that Evil has been depicted as exercising a capacity not just to maim and mutilate but to *silence* its victims, as classically with the raped woman who cannot or will not tell of her ordeal, or (more broadly) with the routine 'unmentionability' of certain taboo diseases in our century, like cancer.

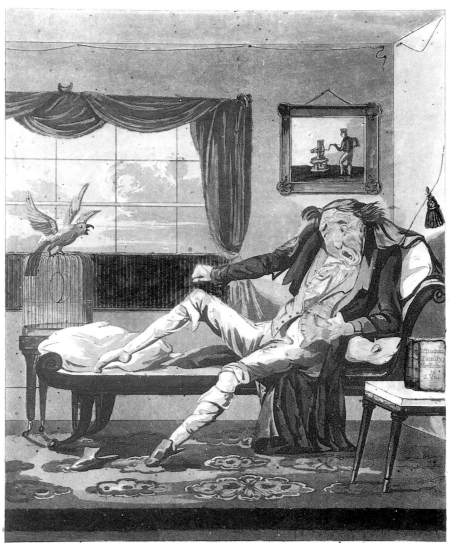

Drawn by M.E. Esq.ʳ   Pubᵈ Augᵗ 1828. by Gillard & Cornish. 48. Strand.

THE CRAMP.

Ecot! it's tied my foot in a Knot — Oh! Oh! O_O_o_o_o

The Cramp. A nineteenth century satirical engraving of a man suffering from a cramp in his leg. (London, Wellcome Institute Library)

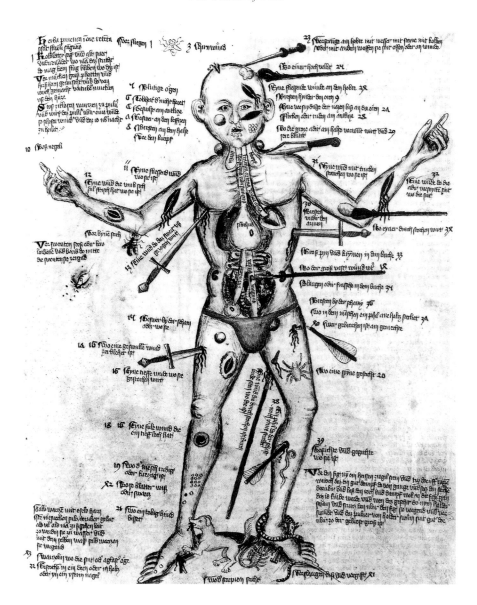

*A Wounded Man: The Apocalypse of St John
in Latin (and German). Fifteenth century.
(London, Wellcome Institute Library)*

Explanations of Pain in Western Culture

To the physician or physiologist, pain has a purpose and a place. It is useful. Philosophically-minded physicians long ago concluded that if, in some negligently-designed Utopia, wounds and frostbite, toxins and infections provoked no pain, survival (individual and racial) would be jeopardised.

Yet if, to the physician, pain has been seen as protective, to the layperson it has been seen as evil, sickening and sinister. Faced with this double vision, philosophers ever since antiquity, have felt obliged to confront the problem of pain, to explain its necessity. One prime aim, for example, of the Epicurean school of Greek thought was to devise a 'damage limitation' philosophy of life, designed to check self-inflicted exposure to pain. A simple life, the Epicureans argued, minimising expectations and ambitions, would offer fewer hostages to fortune. Contrary to the popular stereotype of the sybaritic Epicurean, the good life in their view lay not in the pursuit of hedonism but in the avoidance of heartache. Stoicism similarly taught its followers to soar above passions, appetites and senses, which would only turn to grief.

Western Christian theology took the view that pain was not integral to the initial design of creation. Pain entered the world through original sin and the consequent expulsion from paradise, when God cursed mankind. Man would henceforth be condemned to labour by the sweat of his brow, woman would bring forth in pain, and mankind in general would thereafter suffer disease and death. Thus pain was construed in the Bible as the divine penalty for disobedience, designed to serve as a constant reminder of the turpitude of fallen man. This was a notion reinforced by etymology: 'pain' is derived from *poena*, Latin for 'punishment'.

Down the centuries, preachers further asserted that God visited pain upon the wicked *en masse* in the form of plagues. Furthermore, selected individuals were devoutly to rejoice in affliction as a divinely-ordained cross, in the assur-

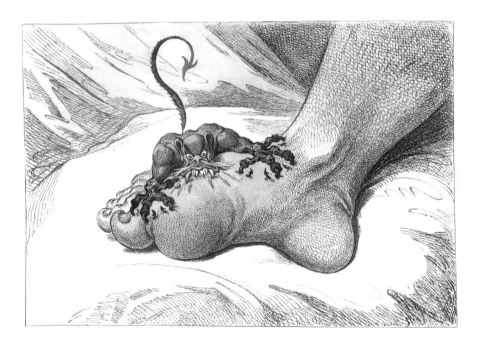

James Gillray *(1757–1815).*
The Gout, 1799.
(London, Wellcome Institute Library)

ance that it formed part of a providential scheme of purificatory tribulation. As Job's trials showed, the proper response to divinely-inflicted suffering was to be, in the literal sense, long-suffering. To be a martyr to disease was no less glorious than to be a martyr to the infidel. Within Catholicism especially, expiatory mortification of the flesh, with goads and hair-shirts or through fasting, struck a blow for holiness, guelled the lusts of the flesh, and emancipated the spirit from the prison-house of the body.

Yet caution was always urged upon Christians, lest they fetishised pain, turning *homo dolorosus*, the man of sorrows, into a vainglorious cult. It was emphasised that charity also required the relief of pain. After all, Luke had been a physician, Christ had performed healing miracles, and finally, heaven promised bliss, not more agony (hell was the place of eternal pain). Hence, Christian apologists developed carefully nuanced positions regarding welfare, charity, and the potential of medicine for a triumph over pain. Suffering, religious moralists stressed, was to be embraced as a gift of Providence, indeed, as a blessing. Yet is was also to be alleviated by medical aid and charitable offices.

These ambiguities, inlaid deep within Christian doctrines towards suffering and ill-health, are echoed, of course, in the casuistry of the churches' attitudes towards war: just wars are holy, but the Christian should also turn the other cheek. The same ambiguities are paralleled in orthodox Christian attitudes towards pain amongst the brute creation: all creatures great and small are God's, yet only humans have immortal souls, hence it is legitimate to inflict a degree of suffering upon animals to meet higher, human needs. Not least, they are found in approaches towards heretics and criminals: apostates may justly be tortured and executed, for the sake of faith and for the greater glory of God.

From medieval times, churchmen and statesmen embraced robust – indeed, we might say, unfeeling – attitudes towards physical pain. Sinful man was bound to be punished, temporally and eternally, by the wrath of God: only the whip and the gallows would preserve the social hierarchy. With the coming of the Age of Reason, philosophers felt obliged to propose rather more refined theodicies. Pain, many writers suggested, should be understood as but a 'partial evil', subserving (as the Augustan poet, Alexander Pope (1688–1744), put it) a 'universal good'. According to Archdeacon Paley's evergreen *Natural Theology* (1802), a perennial Cambridge University student textbook, pain was a 'lesser evil', functional to caution mankind against 'greater' evil. Today's twinge in the toes, Paley thought, is a providential stopsign, directing us to reduce alcohol consumption lest tomorrow we get gout.

Other apologists speculated that God might have brought pain into the world out of a certain creative superfecundity. The existence of the blind, the deaf, the crippled, averred the maverick writer, Soame Jenyns in mid-Georgian England, perhaps enriched creation through the dazzling heterogeneity of types it helped to create. At the very least, such freaks served to

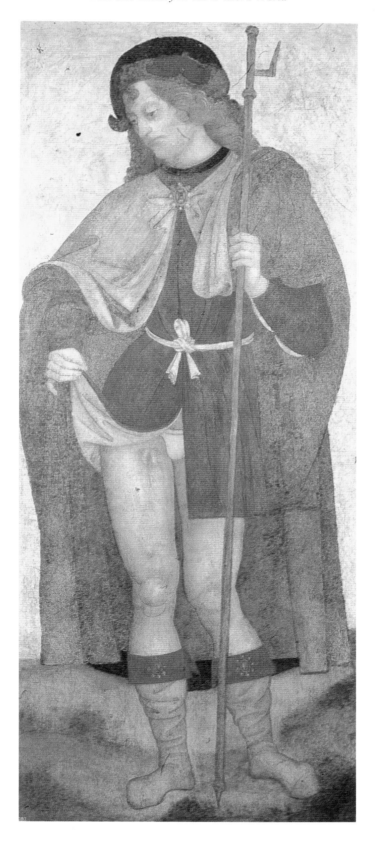

St Roch, Patron of the plague. He is depicted raising the tail of his coat to show a bubo on his thigh. (Anonymous, c. 1500) (London Wellcome Institute Library)

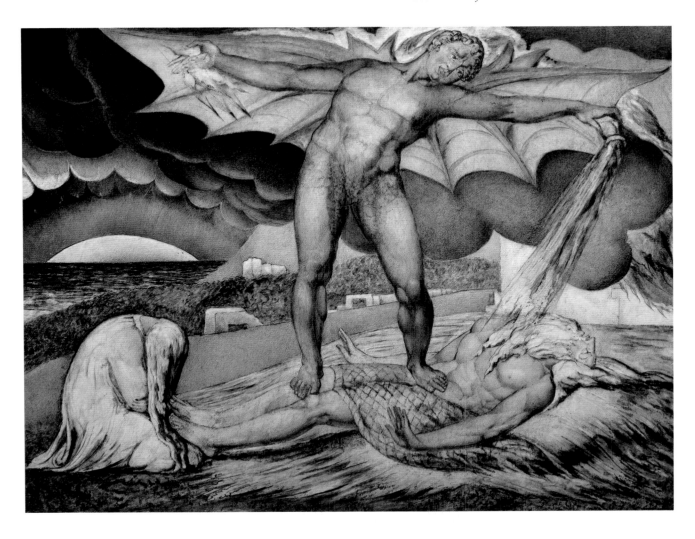

William Blake. Satan inflicting Job with painful abscesses. (c. 1826). (London, Tate Gallery)

fill every step on the chain of being. All that could exist, must necessarily exist: plenitude was aesthetically pleasing to the Supreme Being, even if it entailed some cost through pain.

Down to earth as ever, Samuel Johnson (1709–1784) treated Jenyns' wretched piece of special pleading for pain – the Devil's argument in disguise – with the contempt it deserved. Such apologists for disabilities, Johnson insisted, were tantamount to suggesting that the Almighty took sadistic 'delight in the operations of an asthma, as a human philosopher in the effects of the air pump'; that the higher powers found that swelling 'a man with tympany is as good sport as to blow a frog'; or he chuckled over 'at the vicissitudes of an ague'; and found it 'good sport … to see a man tumble with epilepsy, and revive and tumble again, and all this he knows not why'. It was evil, thought Johnson, to accuse God of being directly to blame for pain. The magnificent sting in the tail is, of course, Johnson's insinuation that Jenyns was vindicating divine justice by proving that God was no more callous in visiting humans with pain, than were people in their own habitual thoughtless cruelties to animals. Johnson admitted, however, that in certain circumstances good could come out of pain: 'The mind is seldom quickened to very vigorous operations but by pain, or the dread of pain.'

Pain in a Secular World: from Explanation to Eradication

The softer sensibilities of the period of the Enlightenment rejected traditional Christianity's apparent acquiescence in the inevitability of pain. Since the eighteenth century, increasingly secular outlooks have given higher priority to the avoidance and elimination of suffering. If medieval thought considered infirmity and misery as endemic features of this vale of tears, modern governments feel obliged to seek the eradication of poverty, disease and deprivation. Medieval Christians fixed their attention on the good death; modern thought seeks the prolongation of painfree life.

In the nineteenth century, the omnipresence of pain became a weapon in the armouries of atheists and agnostics. Pondering the suffering he saw everywhere in the struggle for survival, Charles Darwin (1809-1882) could no longer accept that the wise man automatically looked, as Alexander Pope had recommended, 'from Nature up to Nature's God'.

Christian evolutionists, of course, had their ready riposte. Pain was essen-

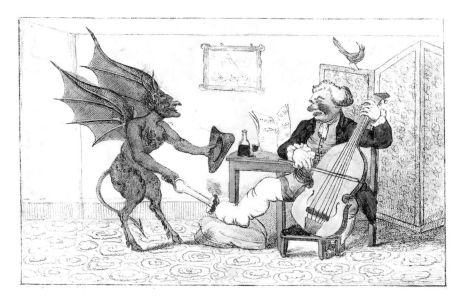

Henry William Bunbury *(1750–1811).*
The Origin of Gout. Engraving showing the
devil applying a burning coal to an infected
foot, 1793. (London, Wellcome Institute
Library)

tial for progress. God, in other words, had programmed the sanction of suffering into the evolutionary process so that the weak would be weeded out, ensuring that none but progressive specimens would survive and thrive. No gain without pain.

For Darwin, the tenents of orthodox Christianity seemed no less brutal than the consequences of the laws of nature. Darwin found he could not stomach the 'cruel' Christian doctrine that unbelievers (there were several in his family) would be condemned to eternal hellfire. His Unitarian contemporary and friend, the economist and novelist Harriet Martineau (1802–1876), was equally scathing in her condemnation of the moral unacceptability of Christian teachings on illness. In her *Life in the Sick-Room: Essays by an Invalid* (1854) she argued that dwelling upon the beauties of suffering cultivated by Evangelicals glamourised morbid self-pity, encouraged wallowing, and sapped the will to be well. Christianity, she thought, made a fetish of pain.

In the secularising shift from the God-centred to the man-centred value system promoted by the Enlightenment, many *philosophes* made the diminution of pain and suffering the keynote of their philosophy, notably, of course, Utilitarians with their *felicific calculus* which aimed to achieve the 'greatest happiness of the greatest number'. The great law reformer, Jeremy Bentham – incidentally an ardent cat-lover – urged an end to wanton cruelty towards animals, not on religious grounds, nor out of any appreciation of animals' rights, but because animals were no less capable of suffering than humans.

Similar arguments applied to debates over the right to suicide. Those who urged the decriminalisation of suicide argued that self-destruction ought to be permissible as a legitimate escape from meaningless and hopeless suffering. The case in the twentieth century for voluntary euthanasia has proceeded along the same lines.

Faced with the puzzle of pain, the medical profession was caught on the horns of dilemma. Many doctors, like the Quakers John Coakley Lettsom (1774–1815) and Thomas Hodgkin (1796–1866), were distinguished for their contributions to humanitarian campaigns against judicial torture, duelling, militarism, the slave trade, imperialism, and other cruel abuses.

On the other hand, medical progress seemed to hinge upon the pursuit of experimental physiology, and in the Victorian era experimentalists suffered attacks from anti-vivisectionist campaigners on account of their seeming indifference to the pain they inflicted upon dumb animals – charges that, of course, are today levied increasingly vociferously by animal rights activists, particularly when experimentation is conducted for lucrative but trivial purposes like cosmetic testing. British doctors and scientists tended to respond to the anti-vivisectionists with a 'greater good' or 'lesser evil' defence, claiming that they were careful to minimise the pain suffered by the animal, by anaesthetising experimental subjects wherever possible, and painlessly destroying them later.

By contrast, certain nineteenth century continental physiologists appeared

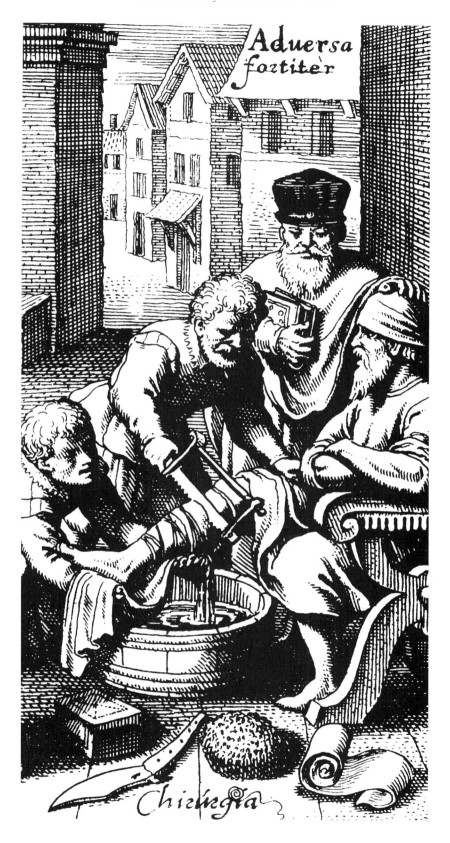

Amputation: detail of a fifteenth century illustration. Excerpt from Severino, M.A. (1580–1656). De efficaci medicina, J. Beyer, Frankfurt, 1646. (London, Wellcome Institute Library)

117

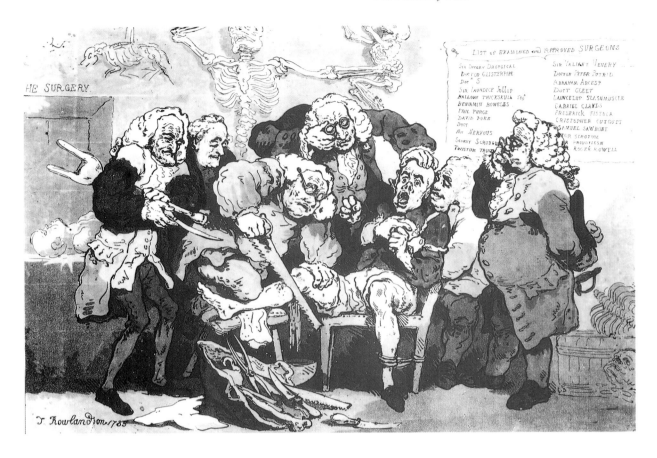

LIST OF EXAMINED AND APPROVED SURGEONS

Sir Dreary Dropsical
Doctor Glisterpipe
Doct S
Sir Iaundice Iullop
Halloon Thickskull Esq
Benjamin Bowels
Paul Purge
David Puke
Doct
Air Nervous
Scurvy Scrubber
Twistum Trunn

Sir Valiant Venery
Doctor Peter Potrid
Abraham Abcess
Doct Gleet
Launcelot Slashmuscle
Gabriel Glands
Frederick Fistula
Cristopher Cutgutt
Samuel Sawbone
Peter Scrotum
Brounperkins
Roger Howell

T. Rowlandson 1785

Thomas Rowlandson
(1756–1827). Amputation, 1793.
(London, Wellcome Institute
Library)

to uphold the Cartesian position on brute sensibilities – animals, they said, were mere automata that could feel nothing – and displayed a certain lofty indifference in the name of science. Since 1876, British legislation has codified procedures for pain control in vivisection experiments.

Conclusion: Pain and Progress

As Robert T. Anderson and Scott T. Anderson show elsewhere in this book, pain clearly differs from culture to culture. But within Western society, has pain changed over *time*? This question has been widely debated. Psychologists and physiologists agree that expectations and circumstances dramatically affect our experience of its intensity. Some have argued that relatively simple epochs, or lower class people in modern society, tend to 'somatise' their complaints, whereas sophisticated cultures and elites 'psychologise' more. Physical events are clearly experienced more or less painfully, according to wider contexts of meaning.

It has often been asserted that the progress of civilisation has augmented sensitivity to pain. This alleged phenomenon could be seen in a positive light.

We might be proud of increasing antipathy to wanton brutality, as evident in campaigns against judicial torture, unnatural punishments and cruel sports. Or we might view it negatively. It could be interpreted as a sapping of hardihood, a deplorable enfeebling of moral fibre and the capacity to bear pain. The eminent Victorian jurist, James Fitzjames Stephen, thus complained in 1860 about such softening: 'that anybody should be in pain and not be immediately relieved – that sharp pain should ever be inflicted upon any one ... shocks and scandalises people in these days.' Stephen feared Britain was becoming 'effeminate'.

These are intractable issues involving many imponderables. Is, for instance, the founding of Amnesty International testimony to the enhanced moral conscience of the twentieth century, or to the fact that torture is currently being employed by more regimes than ever before? Does the use of epidural anaesthetics when women go into labour mark the end, not before time, of a certain punitive streak amongst gynaecologists? Or does it show that Western women have ceased to be prepared to experience their own natural functions?

In any case, direct evidence is utterly inconclusive. Attempts to calibrate degrees of fortitude shown by the sick down the ages alongside some scientific scale of suffering collapse meaninglessly in the teeth of methodological and measuring problems. What is clear is that the human organism has plastic powers of adjustment to meet the challenges demanded of it. Historians are impressed by the habitual bravery of seventeenth and eighteenth century forebears when faced with unanaesthetised amputations, or the prospects of grisly death. But the fortitude seen in a modern field hospital can match it. If less courage is generally shown today by civilian patients, it is probably because less is expected or demanded.

Culture and Pain

Robert T. Anderson and Scott T. Anderson

FROM as far back in time as history records, from the Shang and Zhou dynasties of prehistoric China, from Herodotus who wrote of diverse peoples to the time of Ancient Greece and the cataclysm of two isolated Old Worlds brought together by the voyage of Christopher Columbus, the reality of cultural diversity has impinged on the awareness of thinking people.

Sometimes with reciprocal respect and tolerance for cultural differences – but all too often without – the task has always been, and remains still, to distinguish fact from fiction concerning how people are both alike and different. Recall that Pliny the Elder convinced many Europeans as late as the eighteenth century that in remote parts of the world some people carried their faces like deep relief sculptures on their chests, or faced life with heads like dogs, swishing tails to match. So too, with how humanity copes with pain. People seem to experience pain in different ways, but what do we make of it?

Race and Pain

Pliny described fantasies of racial variability that Romans and later Europeans found fantastic but believable. We still speculate about the nature of racial differences, but hopefully on a more scientific basis. What is the evidence for whether or not races differ in their sensitivity to pain?

Side by side, a European American and an Inuit are helping each other in the Arctic Circle. They work with their hands in ice-cold water for minutes at a time. The European American reports feeling deep pain while the Native Alaskan says nothing. Is this a result of cultural differences? Is the man of Inuit arctic hunting ancestry psychologically tougher? Did he learn as a child that he must be brave? Or do these two men differ physiologically in their capacity to endure the deep pain of ice water?

In this case, the answer is genetic. The anatomy of Eskimo vasculature

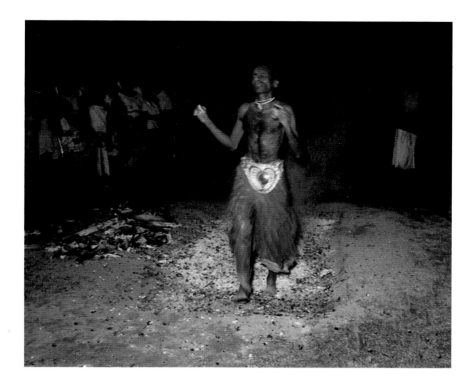

Walking on fire. (Ph. Bury Peerless)

places the arteries carrying warm blood to the hands and fingers closer to the veins returning cooled blood to the body core than is the case for European Americans. Because of the heat exchange that takes place with this anatomic structure, an Inuit man tolerates having his hands in ice water better than a man of different racial origins. The difference is neither psychological nor cultural, it is biological.

A Maring man of the highlands of Papua New Guinea involved in a communal harvest and hunting ritual stands barefoot on stones that have been heating over a fire for more than an hour. Poised on the hot stones, he briefly pierces a piece of fruit with a cassowary bone and then steps away. He shows no evidence of pain. In this case, he is protected by a biological response to a cultural reality. In a society without shoes, his feet are protected by thick, calloused soles. The local European missionary would have suffered a painful burn had he attempted the same feat without shoes. In no way, however, can we detect any distinctiveness in the physiology of pain among the Maring.

One large study that enrolled 40,000 research subjects tested individuals for their tolerance of the deep pain caused by pressure on the Achilles tendon. In that study, at a level that was statistically significant, Whites demonstrated the highest tolerance, Orientals the lowest, with Blacks intermediate. Males in each of the three racial groups tolerated more of this kind of pain than did females in the same groups. Note, however, that it was not a study of pain perception, but of the ability to tolerate the pain. It is possible that the experiment really measured cultural rather than genetic differences. What one person found intolerable, another found merely noticeable. Other experiments indicate that pain sensation declines somewhat with ageing, a finding that is perhaps more solidly based than the last.

What conclusions can we draw? Is it possible that the neurology of pain differs in terms of race, sex and age, but at this time it is not clear that this variability is great, or distinguishes larger populations. For that reason, we will assume that the sensation of pain is essentially the same for all human beings. The important differences in pain experience that we encounter on a world-wide basis must therefore have their explanation in significant differences in cultural attitudes and values.

Feeling Pain: Appearance without Reality

As we set out to explore how people experience pain differently in different contexts, we need to raise a preliminary question: are people always experiencing the pain we think we see?

Fire-walking is practised in India, Java, Europe and America as well as here and there throughout the world. As the ritual is performed by villagers in Greek Macedonia, devotees walk barefoot across a bed of flames with apparent indifference to the intense pain of burning flesh. But appearances are deceptive. They feel some heat, but no pain. This occurs only if they enter the flames too soon, before the incandescent coals become reduced to ashes with so little thermal energy that they will do no damage, or as occurred on at least one occasion, incense thrown into the fire melts, causing hot coals to stick to the skin. Like Pliny's dog-headed people, the pain does not really exist.

In India visitors record in touristic snapshots the apparent indifference to pain of the fakir who sits or lies on a bed of sharp nails. While admittedly no feather bed, it is not exactly the painful instrument of self-torture it appears to be since the body weight is so distributed that very little rests on any one nail. One need only take care not to put too much weight thoughtlessly on one sharp point, to render it relatively painless.

Pain Transformed by Energy

Sometimes a severe pain generator, such as exposure of the body to direct contact with an open flame, is clearly activated, and yet the exposed individual seems to feel the pain as pleasure. Religious ecstasy can make it possible. A classic example in the Western tradition is culled from historical records of witches burned at the stake. Most of the victims unquestionably suffered agonising deaths, but a few are reported to have looked ecstatic as their bodies were cruelly burned. St Joan of Arc is said to have died this way in a state of bliss. We would now assume that an attitude of adoration or self-sacrifice in

opposite page:
Sati, Indian miniature from the Rajput School. With the permission of the Bombay Prince of Wales Museum.
(Ph. Bury Peerless)

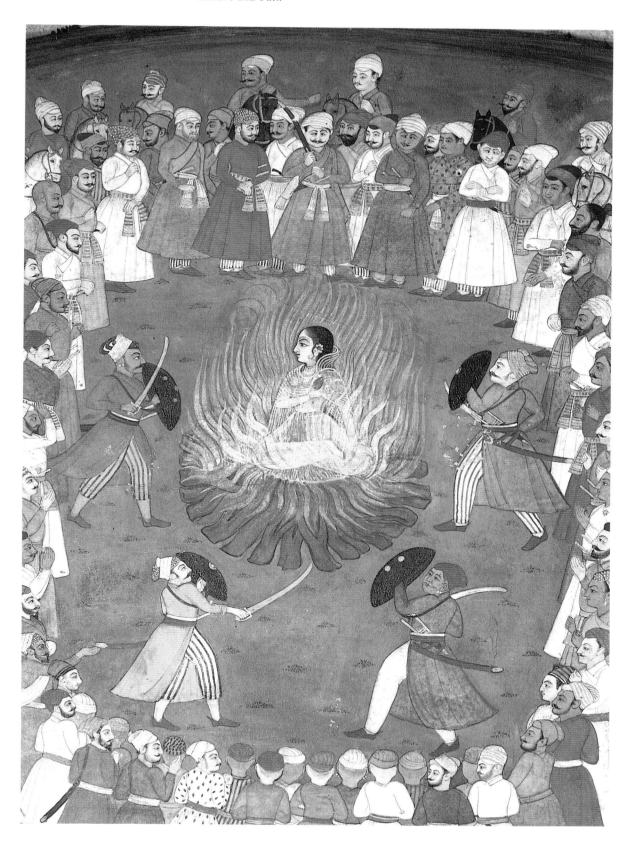

these unusual individuals releases such a rush of endogenous opiates that they experience hypalgesia and euphoria.

The same may be true for the Indian custom of sati, the cremation of living women. The life of a high-caste widow in traditional India was not an easy one. Often a young woman, even a teenager, would be forced from the time of her husband's death to sleep on the ground, wear drab clothes, subsist on one single saltless meal a day and spend her days in pious ritual. Since her mere presence brought bad luck, she was not welcome at family festivals, which were the highlights of traditional social recreation. Shunned and hidden away, she lived out the remaining decades of her life as a closely guarded prisoner. Her parents-in-law supervised her every move, worried that her slightest sensual dalliance might threaten the eternal well-being of their deceased son. Is it surprising then, that in such times a woman might willingly mount the cremation pyre to burn as a companion to the corpse of her husband?

Self-immolation changed a widow's prospects smartly, since it ensured that she and her husband would enjoy thirty-five million years of heavenly delight. The custom of widow immolation was old in certain parts of Asia. It was known to the ruling families of Sumeria and of ancient China. In India, despite efforts to extinguish the practice, it occurs even today as a newsworthy item of speculation. Did she throw herself willingly on the funeral pyre, or was she forced upon it? Without question, sati often brought a painful death but it was stoically endured. At other times, however, it might have been experienced as an ecstasy of transcendental release.

Many other examples of a euphoric pain experience are seeded throughout the ethnographic and historic literature. They include from time to time the account of a dedicated protester in Southeast Asia, suicidally soaked in petrol, who calmly self-ignites while seated Buddha-like in a meditational pose. His grievance, embodied and inflamed, is witnessed by millions as it is carried live be television. He may be brave and stoic, but in some cases at least, we suspect that a transcendal state is achieved.

Ecstatic dying is believed to have characterised thousands of Aztec men at a time, the losers of ancient Middle American wars. Called Battles of the Flowers, they were not fought for booty or territory, but to obtain young bodies as sacrifices. The losers became the winners, in a sense, transformed into heroes who would shortly mount steep pyramids where their last conscious awareness would be that of the priest cutting jaggedly into their chests with a black flint knife to roughly snatch out hearts honoured to provide pulsating gifts for the gods. Ceramic effigies of these sacrificial youths show faces aglow in serene acceptance.

A last example must suffice. An old custom was witnessed a few years ago by an archaeologist searching in remote regions of the Deccan plateau of South Asia for survivals of a once widespread but now nearly extinct custom. It requires a man to undergo a very painful procedure. Having volunteered, he is ritually bathed, dressed in red silk trousers and turban, covered with garlands

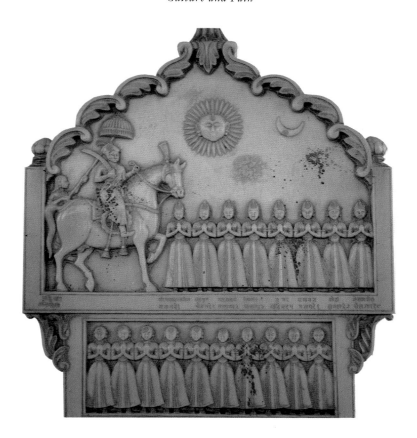

Sati memorial showing the Queen Mother of Rajput on horseback, headed for her ritual suicide on the funeral pyre of one of the Maharajas of Bikaner. On the same memorial, eighteen queens of lower social status or concubines escort her to her death. (Ph. Bury Peerless)

of flowers and declared to be a deity incarnate, a god for the day. The devotee appears to be quite unconcerned when the village carpenter thrusts a large steel hook under the skin of his lower back, and then a second one next to the first. With ropes attached to the hooks, a wooden beam hoists the celebrant into the sky, from where he imparts his blessings to children and fields. In the past after the still customary goat sacrifices were offered, he would have had his head cut off and placed on display, but that part of the custom no longer takes place. Throughout the ceremony, it is reported, the hook swinger experiences a state of exaltation, showing no sign whatsoever of suffering pain.

It must be acknowledged that pain was possibly dulled in some of the above cases by herbal analgesics, since we know that opioids were widely available in Asia. Almost without question, Aztec sacrificial warriors were helped along by the ingestion of hallucinogens. Nonetheless, it is abundantly clear that religious ecstasy alone is capable of masking enormous pain.

Trance and Pain

On the island of Bali, temple dancers choreographed by old traditions gyrate around a frightening impersonation/incarnation of Rangda the witch. In an instant they fall into a deep trance. In this altered state of consciousness they move stiffly, predictably, attacking the hideous Rangda when she turns her back on them, but falling in stiff seizures on the ground at her mere backwards glance. Suddenly the dance warriors fragment into individual pirouettes, each man stabbing endlessly at his own chest with his curved steel dagger, falling to the ground in a paroxysm of masochistic energy. That man later will recall no pain and will suffer no damage to the skin.

The Balinese dancer is in a trance so akin to religious ecstasy that the states of consciousness may well be psychodynamically and biochemically identical. Yet trance seems different in one important way. It is induced by participation

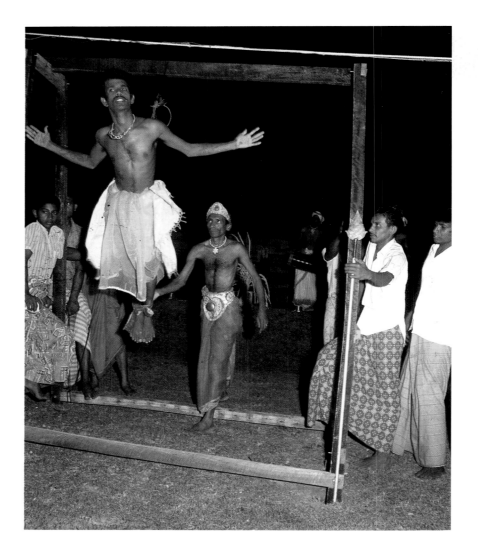

Levitation ceremony, Kataragama, Sri Lanka. A man with hooks in his back is swinging freely in the air and giving blessings. (Ph. Bury Peerless)

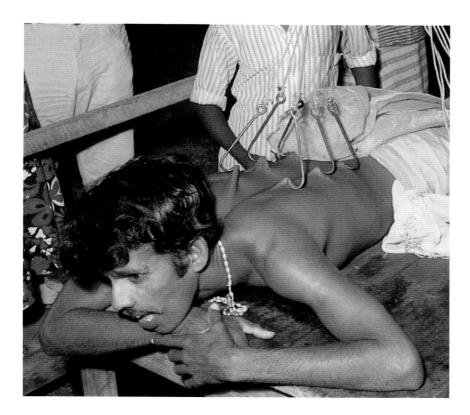

Levitation ceremony, Kataragama, Sri Lanka. Metal hooks are being inserted in the back of a man preparing for the ceremony. (Ph. Bury Peerless)

in the dance, a recurrent, planned activity, that occurs simultaneously to a dozen men at once. Trance induction is clearly a culturally shaped way of altering consciousness that can render the individual insensitive to pain.

Trance against pain need not take place only in a religious context. We recently examined the photographic and statistical records of an American physician who performs painful reconstructive surgery to repair severe burn wounds. In select cases he relies solely on hypnosis for pain control. To this end he spends hours with each patient, far more than busy surgeons usually provide. His payoff comes, however, at the moment of the operation, when he needs only to whisper in the patient's ear and the most painful debridement or plastic surgery can be performed with none of the untoward effects of chemical anaesthesia. The pain is there, but the patient has no awareness of it.

Our most recent documentation of trance-induced insensitivity to pain took place in South America. We were in Northeastern Brazil with Professor Sidney Greenfield to document operations in which the healer performs cold knife surgery without the use of anaesthetics and with a defiant disregard for sterile technique. Let us take just one example of the hundreds of cases we observed.

Ms Prado, a young woman in her twenties, made her way by overnight bus to the healing centre in which a middle-aged man, Joao de Abadiania, personally and individually treats hundreds of patients on each of three days a week.

The overwhelming majority receive only a scribbled prescription for bottles of medicine as they shuffle past the healer on the throne-like chair. A select few become candidates for surgery.

We were unable to determine what medical or psychological problem troubled Ms Prado so much that she had made this pilgrimage, because we first saw her as she appeared in the auditorium facing an intent audience of several hundred who had been singing and praying that morning while they waited for the scheduled two to six surgeries to be performed as spiritual theatre.

Standing against the wall, facing the audience with her eyes closed, Ms Prado was gently guided to a stool where she remained impassive as Joao selected a steak knife from an unsterile tray of otherwise standard surgical instruments. Holding her eye open with his left hand, he gently but firmly scraped the edge of the knife repeatedly across the cornea, sclera and inner lid until he had accumulated a thin layer of fluid or debris on the knife which he then wiped cavalierly on her blouse. The corneal reflex, normally instantaneous was deadened. She felt no pain, she later told us in the recovery room.

Without pausing, Ms Prado arose and was guided back against the wall, standing with no apparent tendency to faint, as Joao slowly and deliberately pushed her clothing aside to expose the lower abdomen. Selecting a scalpel

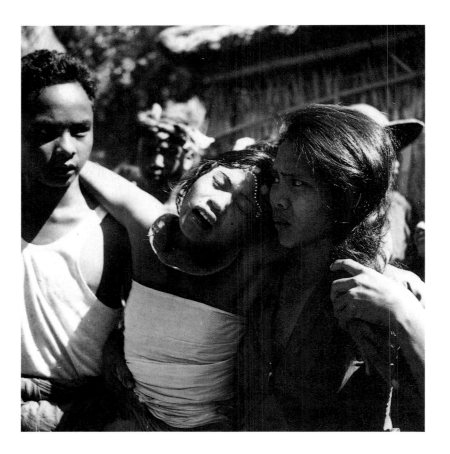

Barung (Kris) dance: Pain under hypnosis.
A dancer in a trance, South Bali, Indonesia.
(Ph. Theo Meier 1940–42)
(Museum für Volkekunde, Basel)

from his tray, he methodically performed an eight centimetre incision, probed deeply into it with his bare finger, still covered with blood from an earlier patient, and then sutured the wound using an upholstery needle and thread. Again, she experienced absolutely no pain.

Then a third procedure was performed as the instrument tray provided a straight pliers-like haemostat with which he grasped a small amount of cotton. Tilting her chin up by leverage with his left hand against her forehead, he touched the tip of the ten centimetre steel implement momentarily to one nostril, and then in a deliberate manner thrust it straight into her head reaching the hilt. Not yet finished, he took hold of the handles with his fingers against the palm of his hand and roughly twisted it several complete rotations clockwise. The worst over, he finally pushed her chin smoothly to her chest, withdrew the haemostat and permitted a fulsome stream of blood to flow onto clothes already wet with blood from her abdominal surgery. Again she felt no pain, merely the sensation of something going into her nose.

Ms Prado's case illustrates a form of pain relief that can be encountered in many parts of the world. She went through a clearly identifiable induction procedure before she entered the surgical theatre. Surrounded by a score of entranced mediums in the sanctified space of a nearby room, one faced her while another stood behind. The two gently pushed her back and forth until she began spontaneously to rock rhythmically on her own, her eyes staring vacantly into eternal space. She had fallen into a deep trance.

The patient was under deep hypnosis, but she was not the only one. Earlier in the morning, while praying in anguish before a small altar, Joao was

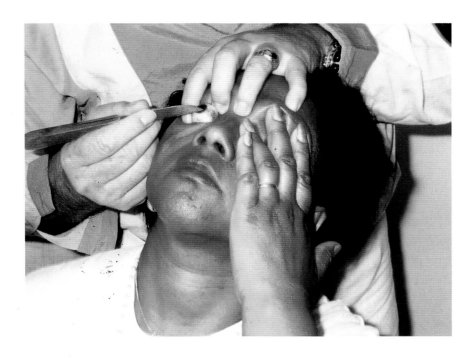

Ms Prado treated by Joao of Abadiana, Brazil, 1992. (Ph. Scott Anderson, M.D.)

suddenly possessed by the essence of Saint Ignatius of Loyola. A team of mediums joined him outside his private chambers and they too fell into trances. Everyone involved was in an altered state of consciousness as Ms Prado demonstrated her remarkable insensitivity to pain and emotional stress.

Feeling Pain with Indifference

Joao usually performs surgery only on a select few who appear to submit while in deep trance. Occasionally, however, Joao operates on a patient who is not in an altered state of consciousness, yet who appears not to feel significant pain. The abdominal incision, probe and suturing performed on Ms Prado was witnessed several times on others when pain control would seem better described as a placebo response than as a product of hypnotic suggestion. In these instances, patients were convinced the operation was beneficial, and that belief alone appears to have provided a beneficial response, protection against pain.

This is seen most clearly in the high-volume practice of Antonio de Oliveria, who was a bricklayer by trade until he began to incorporate the spirit of Dr Ricardo, a long dead physician. It is quite astonishing to see this aggressive village artisan cut a ten to twelve centimetres incision deeply into a patient's abdomen, penetrating four to five centimetres through skin and into fatty tissue while the patient merely raises his head to look quizzically at the wound and at the audience. Later, the same patient chatted amicably with Antonio's young wife. The man seemed completely at ease, not so much indifferent to pain as unaware of it. It seems clear that when the cultural context of cutting and penetrating the body is quite devoid of fear, the mere absence of fear can be protective. It is a reminder that pain can be separated from suffering. When anxiety and fear are removed, pain can become tolerable.

Culture and Stoicism

In a more urban part of Brazil, Mauricio Megalhaes cuts or needles each of several hundred patients in a row during any single evening when he is possessed by the spirit of Dr Adolf Fritz. Dr Fritz was a German physician who died during World War I. Thought to have been responsible for evil acts performed as a military doctor during the dictatorship of Kaiser Wilhelm, Dr Fritz is still working off bad karma. Because he possesses no body of his own, he uses Mauricio's as a way to practice beneficial surgery in our time. It does not matter that Mauricio never advanced in elementary school beyond the fourth year.

The induction in Mauricio's clinics is carried out by indirect means: responding to individual conferences with devotees, sitting and listening to monotone lectures on spirituality, singing repetitive Christian songs, and then standing in a line that advances slowly and reverently towards the charismatic surgeon, results in the mass hypnotising of a whole room of patients.

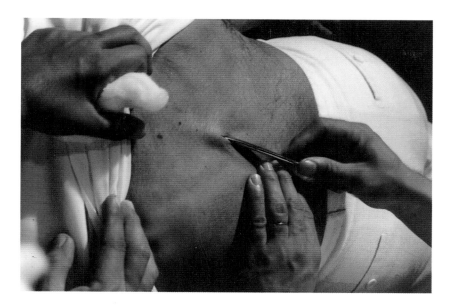

Mr Barreto during surgery on his spine
performed by Mauricio.
(Dr Fritz) Brazil, 1992.
(Ph. Scott Anderson, M.D.)

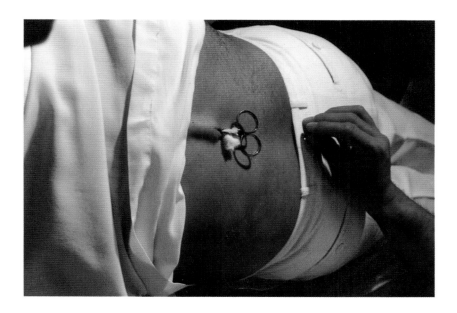

Mr Barreto during surgery on his spine by
Mauricio (Dr Fritz) Brazil, 1992.
(Ph. Scott Anderson, M.D.)

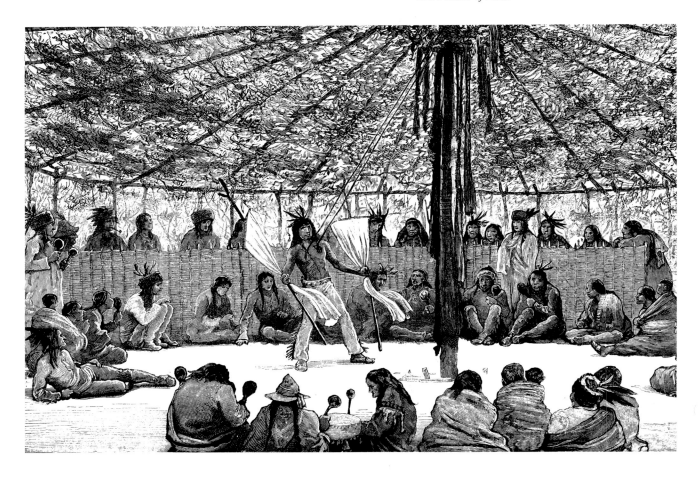

Dance of the Sun. Engraving showing the Cree Indian initiation ceremony, N.W. of Canada, 1886. (Mary Evans Picture Library)

Mauricio performs the surgery rapidly, moving unhesitant back and forth between two surgical setups positioned side by side so that he is not delayed by the few moments it takes for patients to get on and off tables. We found that hypnotic control of pain and/or lack of fear worked better for some than others in this assembly line approach to surgery.

Some experienced no pain relief at all and were merely stoic. Mr Barreto who is seventy-eight years old, provides an example of hypnotic failure. This fearful, retired gentleman suffered from occasional, recurrent low back pain with some numbness in his right leg. The pain and numbness, mild to moderate in intensity, always improved substantially with chiropractic treatment. He had recently moved to Brazil, however, where he was out of touch with his chiropractor. He came to Mauricio as an alternative health care provider.

Mr Barreto submitted to some brutal surgery. First, by means of a scalpel, a five centimetre vertical incision was made centrally in the mid back area, quite distant from the area of low spinal pathology. Then, using the incision as an entry cut, a blunt-ended, closed haemostat was forced under the skin against considerable tissue resistance until it penetrated fifteen centimetres up the back between the shoulder blades, leaving only its scissors-like handles exposed. A woman in street clothes, to her utter surprise, was commanded to grasp the handles and pull out the instrument. Using all of her strength, she provided a clear demonstration of how much brute force the penetration had required. In an answer to a follow-up questionnaire filled out one month later, Mr Barreto stated that the pain of the surgery was the most excruciating pain he could possibly imagine. Yet at the time he showed no sign of it at all. He was stoic.

In other societies, where warriors are heroes, Mr Barreto's sort of bravery constitutes a highest virtue. In the US among the Plains Indians of a century ago, the ability to endure hunger, thirst, cold, heat, fatigue and great pain was celebrated in the annual Sun Dance. The central feature of the ceremony was a mass ordeal by young men, most of whom simply danced for a number of days, while looking towards the sun, as a self-induced trial of fortitude. However, the truly great warrior tortured himself in a manner that resembled the ordeal of hook-hangers on the other side of the world in India.

The Sun Dancer attached himself to one or more long cords by passing them through pierced folds of skin on his back, shoulders or chest. Attached to heavy buffalo skulls, he danced around the centre pole, tugging on the heavy, reluctant skulls until one by one, the cords tore through his flesh to release him. The similarity of the Indian and Amerindian culture trait – tearing against pierced folds of skin by attachment to ropes – dramatises the power of a culture to shape responses to pain. The Indian hook-hanger escaped pain through religious ecstasy. The Native American, also pursuing sacred goals, celebrated his pain very differently as a badge of fortitude; he was intensely stoic.

Rites of passage are the common arena for demonstrating a stoic endurance to pain. We think of a Nuer boy, just eleven years old, in an East African community of warrior cattle herders. When a boy is old enough he must acquire three deep cuts from ear to ear across the skin of his forehead. They will heal as raised keloid scars that mark him as no longer a child, but a man who can join other young warriors in amorous and military exploits. They entitle him eventually to marry and become a father. From the time he was a toddler, he has looked forward to acquiring these marks of manly status.

The man who does the cutting carries several much used steel blades in a hollowed wooden purse. The knives are laid out in the dust to be available as needed. The naked boy, still too young for pubic hair, lies quietly on his back, his head resting on a scooped out mound of sand that will collect a pool of blood as the surgery proceeds. Without a word, the lad crosses his arms on his chest and then remains completely immobile. The cutting proceeds slowly, the blade tugging against resistant flesh, each cut beginning at the midline and moving towards one side or the other until six slow pain cuts have been completed. No more than a momentary wince and two small puddled tears at the corner of each eye suggest for a brief instant the existence of a sensation of sharp cutting pain manfully subdued.

Boys are not required to be so brave about pain everywhere. A Hausa boy in another part of Africa is supposed to show his courage when circumcised. He is made to sit, stark naked, with his legs spread apart so that his penis is exposed over a hole in the ground that will catch his blood. While firmly held from behind in the arms of an assistant, he faces the circumciser who cuts away the foreskin in five or six painful strokes. The boy writhes against restraint and cries out *'Wayyo Allah! Wayyo Allah!'*, the Hausa equivalent of 'Oh God, that hurts! Oh God, that hurts!'.

In the village of Kanganaman, Papuan New Guinea boys are supposed to remain stoically silent while from their necks to their knees their skin is cut with razor blades in an all-day ordeal. Loud drumming masks their poorly restrained cries of pain and anguish.

Deep in the Brazilian rainforest a completely terrorised Kaingang boy has his lip pierced. The operator struggles to twist and turn a decorative plug that must be inserted while the blood flows. The toddler howls, his mother weeps, and that is all right.

Female rites of passage may also include painful experiences. Young Nuer women are equally as stoic as Nuer boys. They submit calmly to a procedure of using the sharp point of a pin to lift a small piece of skin that is then cut away with a razor blade. Laughing and talking as the operation proceeds, scores of these painful cuts create geometric patterns to cover much of the upper torso. The cuts will heal as permanent ornamental scars. The cutting is very painful, but no one seems to notice.

Stoicism in women in many societies is a demand of childbirth. Nisa, an Ikung San woman of South Africa, experienced what she described as unbearable pain when she gave birth to a child. Some women cry, she recalled, but she did not. When her contractions signalled that parturition was at hand, she quietly walked away from her companions to deliver herself alone in complete silence at the base of a tree. The ordeal over, her woman companions came running only when they heard the baby cry.

Among the rural women of Greece, to cry out during childbirth is equated with displaying no sexual shame. Often a woman will bite a blanket during delivery as a way to suppress the urge to scream. To quiet her urge to shout, one woman bit her lips until they were running with blood. Only the women assisting her in the birthing room were allowed to hear her stifled groans. To the wider world, the labouring room was a place of silence and womanly pride.

The Meaning of Stoicism

We have documented a stoic quiescence for men, women and children in many parts of the world, but it must be noted that the emotions and thoughts lying behind stoicism can be quite variable. In a classic study of responses to pain among patients in a veteran's hospital in New York (carried out from 1951 to 1954), Mark Zborowski, an anthropologist, found that both Old American and Irish-American patients accepted pain without complaint.

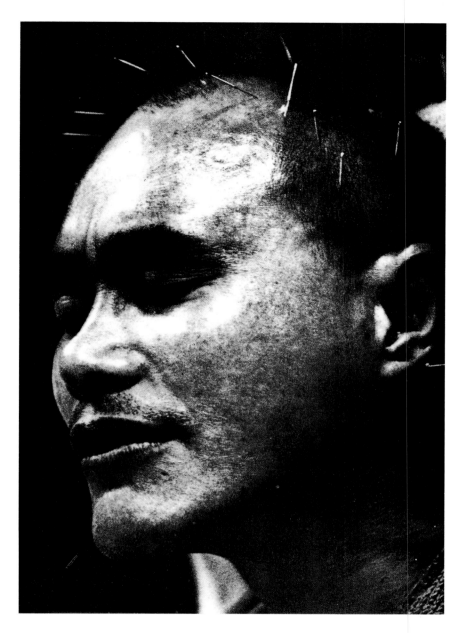

Acupuncture. La Médecine Chinoise, by
George Beau. (Paris, Editions du Seuil, 1965)

However they differed greatly in how they experienced the meaning of pain.

To understand the pain behaviour of the Old American, we need to distinguish private from public pain. In private, an Old American may have collapsed into tears, but never in public. The Old American tended, therefore, to withdraw in the face of strong pain. In the hands of doctors and nurses, however, to admit to pain was permitted because the professional situation transformed complaints into purposeful discussion. Possessing a mechanistic attitude to the body and its functions, the Old American had considerable faith in the abilities of doctors, and tended therefore to be fairly optimistic about ultimate outcomes.

Irish-American patients, equally uncomplaining when in pain, differed from Old Americans in how they felt about their sickness. They lacked the optimism of Old Americans. In public, an Irish patient masked his pain. He was scarcely more vocal in a medical context. These patients articulated pain concerns very ineptly, despite displays of loquacious skill under other circumstances. The Irish-American felt helpless, guilty about becoming ill and very pessimistic about the future.

Zborowski also described two kinds of patient who were the very opposite of stoics. In his research he demonstrated that Italian-American and Jewish-American veterans tended to display highly emotional responses to pain. They groaned and cried. They complained. They laid in wait to provide any and all a description in redundant detail of how they suffered. They shared a cultural train that permitted vivid expressions of pain, yet their pain behaviour rested on very different emotional foundations.

The Jewish patient tended to experience a future-oriented anxiety. Pain was taken as a frightening warning of ultimate possible doom. This patient needed reassurance from the doctor, who found it almost impossible to evade listening to a recital of complaints that seemed endless. But this patient was sceptical toward the doctor. He was reluctant to take prescribed medications. He worried that the pills might only provide temporary improvement at the cost of disguising symptoms in a way that could mislead his physician. He also feared becoming addicted to pain-killing drugs. In his pain and suffering, it was his suffering that overwhelmed him.

The Italian-American was equally vocal when in pain. In place of scepticism however, this patient showed great trust in doctors and hospitals. In place of a Jewish future orientation, the Italian experienced a present-oriented apprehension. His focus was on the pain as such. In complete trust, he accepted, indeed begged, for strong analgesics to quiet the pain. As soon as the pain was gone he became calm, full of smiles, and almost forgetful of the illness.

The work of Zborowski was carried out half a century ago. To the extent that we would set different standards to for this kind of research in our time, his characterisations resemble stereotypes rather than documented generalisations. We would want more precision about the nature and quality of the pain, we would want assessments to be blinded in order to remove bias in interpretation, we would ask for a clearer definition of ethnicity, since some of these veterans were third-generation Americans. In spite of these questions, however, Zborowski's generalisations were consistent with his anecdotal experience of many Americans nurses and physicians.

Based on these findings, Zborowski convincingly made one important point. Not only does culture shape the way in which people communicate their discomfort and unhappiness, it also shapes how pain can be associated with powerful existential concerns and with ultimate eschatological issues.

The sensation of pain is a biological given, essentially the same for every normal individual. The experience of pain, however, is shaped by families and societies. This aspect of pain can vary enormously, ranging from painful ecstasy, through placebo- and trance-induced unawareness, to brave stoicism and unbridled histrionics. To think about pain solely as a biomedical, physiological phenomenon is to neglect its most important dimensions.

Culture and the Treatment of Pain

Just as societies differ in how they react to the experience of pain, they also differ in how they seek relief. Efforts at palliation are enormously diverse. In Asia, many forms of pain are treated by acupuncture, cupping, poultices, massage and herbs. Needling techniques may be effective as counter-irritants, by blocking nerve transmission (the gating mechanism) or by inducing the release of endorphins. In cupping for pain one lights a flame in a glass or cup to create a vacuum so that the vessel will attach to the skin and elevate a circle of skin. In wet cupping, small incisions are made before application. The vacuum draws blood into the vessel when it is attached. The major benefit of cupping is as a counter-irritant. Poultices stimulate local blood circulation which may help to remove noxious chemicals. They function simultaneously as counter-irritants. Massage also improves circulation and serves as a counter-irritant. Herbs may contain pain-reducing chemicals.

In other parts of the world cupping, poultices, massage and herbs are widely used. Among the many ethnic groups of New Guinea the favoured form of

Ants' headband: a strip of woven palm tree leaves on which a few bees and ants are placed. The headband is applied to the forehead to treat migraines. It can also be applied to any other part of the body where pain is experienced. French Guiana, Waiyama Indians. (Pitt Rivers Museum, Oxford)

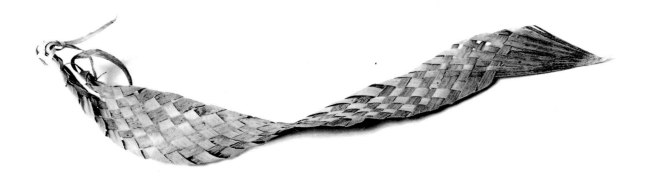

counter-irritation is to apply stinging nettles to the body. Throughout Eurasia and the Americas, many kinds of pain are palliated in sweat baths. Herbs are used in every major region of the world. High in the Andes, underfed Indians numb the hunger of pain and aching bodies by chewing coca leaves to achieve a mild form of narcotic relief. Beer, mead, wine and distilled liquors are reported for pain relief in many parts of the world, even though their efficacy for this purpose is limited.

Until the development of modern pharmaceuticals, traditional efforts to treat the sensation of pain on the whole were largely ineffective. However, there is more to the experience of pain than nerve sensations. From a world-wide perspective, pain is most commonly treated by shamans who perform sacred healing rituals. Shamans do very little to treat the sensation of pain, but a lot to treat suffering associated with pain.

In the village of Huautla de Jimenez high in the mountains of Mexico, a Mazatec Indian shaman treats a young woman's recurrent headaches by employing a variety of ritual techniques. During the preceding four days her patient has purified herself by sexual abstinence and prayer. In the shaman's humble house, chants and supplications are pronounced before an altar on which pictures of Catholic saints are embraced by flowers and copal incense, ritual items known to pre-Columbian Aztecs. With only the light of the altar candle, an unbroken egg is passed over the young woman's forehead. It is believed to absorb some of the sickness. It will rest on the altar until it is passed over her body again later in the evening. Medicinal herbs ground into a green powder are rubbed into her hair and onto her arms, back and neck. The powder, too, is thought to have curative value. Finally the time arrives for both the shaman and her patient reverently to consume a small bowl filled with morsels of an hallucinogenic mushroom. After chewing and swallowing, the candle is extinguished, and in total darkness during the long hours of the night they experience visions and discuss the wisdom they contain.

Does this kind of cure work? It may well be effective. The lesson that may be learned from the above is that much of the experience of pain is not the sensation as such, but the experience in a larger sense. Rituals may trigger biochemical responses that lessen the sensation of pain but above all permit the patient to cope better with personal and social issues. Ritual can help to alleviate the suffering associated with pain. We should never underestimate the value of these symbolic measures for relieving anxieties and reducing and calming emotions.

Pain, in summary, does not occur in mindless bodies. It occurs in the context of cultures which vary greatly in how they shape the experience. People feel and communicate their pain in diverse ways that cannot be explained in simple physiological terms. Concomitantly, they treat pain in complex ways that may produce great satisfaction, even if the treatment does not remove the painful sensation itself. One important part of the puzzle of pain is that it occurs as a product of one's culture.

On Pain, in Brief

Michel Enaudeau

WHEN the philosopher speaks of pain, he or she also speaks of pleasure. It does not mean that he or she is less capable than the historian of discerning, distinguishing and discriminating. It means that the philosopher, probably similar to the physiologist, is first and foremost guided by sensation – if not the simplest or the least complex, – at least the ordinary type of sensation: 'In my leg, because of the chain, there was the painful and now it is the pleasant that

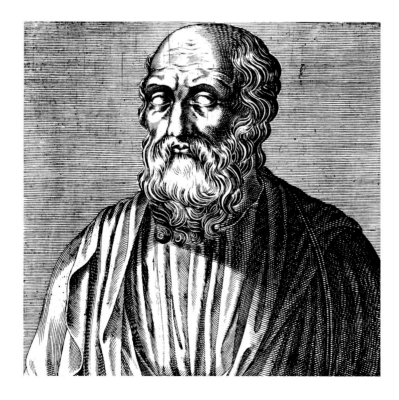

Plato, Greek philosopher
427–347 AD.
(Mary Evans Picture Library)

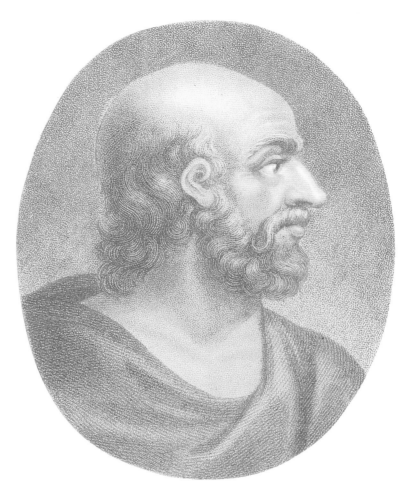

Hippocrates, Greek doctor 460–377 AD.
Reproduction of a stone belonging to
J. Tassie by J. Chapman.
(Mary Evans Picture Library)

seems to come next.'[1] So Socrates said on the day before his death while untied for a moment.

These few words represent the dominant direction to be found in philosophy – from the Greeks to Freud – if we limit ourselves to the writings of the latter prior to *Beyond the Pleasure Principle*. The recurrent idea, like a theme and its variations, is that pain comes first and pleasure derives from it while pain is progressively ceasing. The absence of painful or disagreeable sensation is equivalent to a kind of sensory neutrality, the positive naming of which is pleasure. In this progressive change from pain to pleasure, the mind perceives the restoration of a balance or an order that pain threatens, shatters and destroys. Hence, Lucretius' statement: 'Pain emerges as soon as the elements of matter, thrown into confusion by some force through the living flesh and the limbs, become agitated in the chaos of their abode ... but when everything returns to normal, it is sweet pleasure that follows.'[2] And in Epicurus' words:

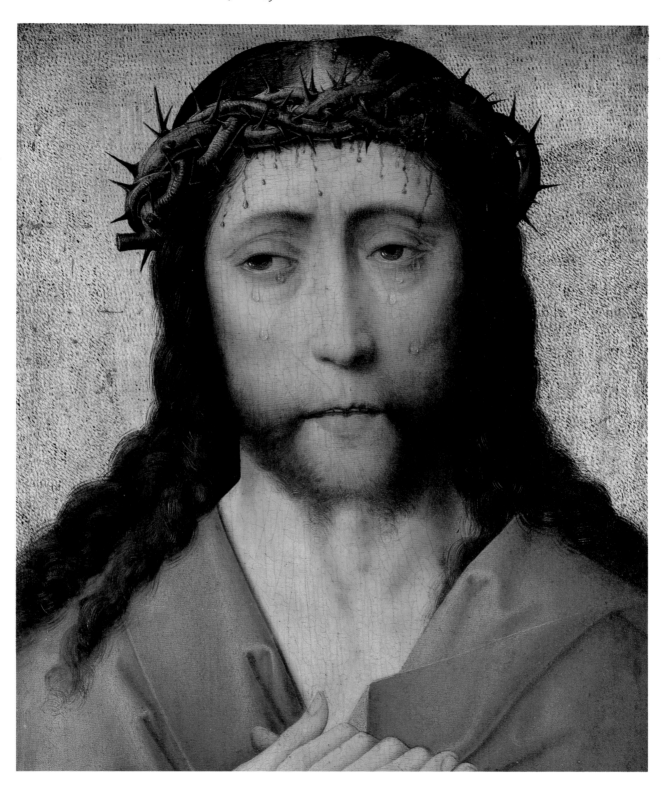

Bouts. *Christ crowned with thorns.*
(The National Gallery, London)

'It [nature] is in fact preserved through pleasure, but destroyed through pain.'[3] Isn't this the same idea, improved by medical science, that guides Bergson much later? Pain is an effort that fails to 'pull things back together'. The impotence of pain is commensurate to the inadequacy of the localised effort it represents: the organism is a whole, only sensitive to combined effects.[4] From pain approached through sensation to the vanity of what Bergson calls pain/effort, it is the disparity of the heterogeneous proximity of pain/pleasure which asserts itself. Enjoyment is the feeling of the promotion of life whereas pain is a hindrance to life.[5]

As far as it is grasped apart from pleasure, as far as it is conquered, pain generates a sort of displacement. More important than pain itself is its mastery and domination. In the Western world, for example, the two are embodied in the figure of the wise man, which is different from that of the philosopher. The wise man proves able to face and endure the ordeal of cruelty and torture. Seneca enlarges on examples of this kind. The endurance of pain is a prerequisite to happiness (Epicurus).

Pain as a relationship of the self to the self is 'good' as long as it brings something, as long as it gives access. Let us listen to the still vivid echo of this in the

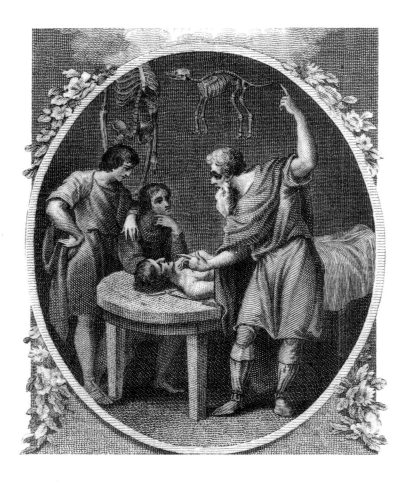

Claude Galen, Roman doctor. Evidence of Christian religion. Drawing by R. Corbould and engraved by C. Warren. (Mary Evans Picture Library)

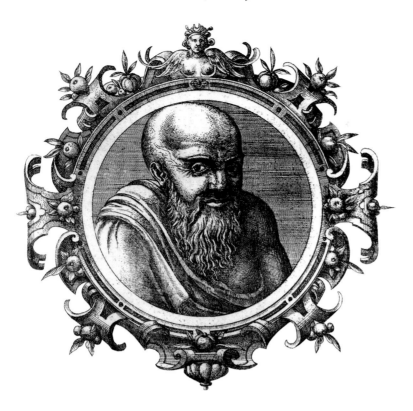

Socrates, Athenian philosopher 470–399 AD.
(Mary Evans Picture Library)

words of a contemporary writer: 'this pain gave me extraordinary strength, it made me a colossus, a giant, not because of my endurance but because it became an instrument of self-discovery which raised my idea of myself.'[6]

Pain is a transition, a change from one condition to another. In the famous allegory of the cave, the progression from delusion toward knowledge does not occur without bruising. Plato, of course, is not ignorant of the suffering which goes with the ascent toward the opening of the cave, toward the light of truth.[7] Thus pain commutes from an intellectual, social and ethical order into another order, different if not superior to the one which is left behind. It commutes one condition. This commutation happens to be both individual and collective, as is achieved by the initiatory rites performed by societies studied by the ethnologist.[8] From this point of view, pain is perceived as a propaedeutics, as a 'paideia'. It initiates, introduces, educates: it makes an adult out of a child, a wise man out of a man. In short, it converts. And this power of conversion is an extravagant feature of pain.

Can philosophy go further? Can we say about pleasure, as Descartes did about the finite – in spite of what is conveyed by language, can we say that it is not the first, positive term, the negative aspect of which would be displeasure? On the contrary one must have an idea of the infinite in order to think one's

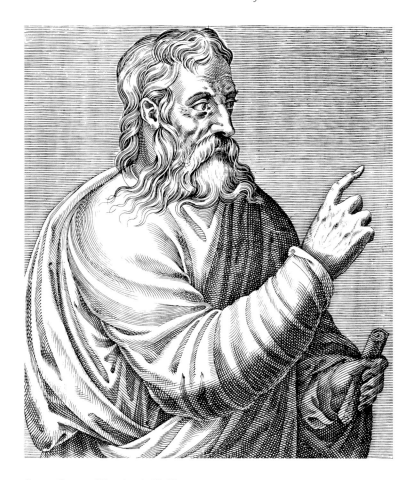

Seneca, Roman philosopher 4–65 AD.
(Mary Evans Picture Library)

own limits; just the same, one must have felt pain in order to feel pleasure. When he decides to call displeasure 'negative pleasure', Kant places 'the disposition of the mind [to seize] something out of the opposition of the two sensations.'[9]

The German philosopher stresses the logical relationship that the example of psychology provides. Kant, as a critical philosopher, makes pleasure and pain (displeasure), as a feeling, the touchstone of the aesthetic judgement. And if there is pure pleasure, it is the feeling originated by the beautiful, i.e. the feeling produced by the free play of understanding and imagination which is revealed by the ability to judge. This 'purity' is unknown to displeasure. The feeling within which pain is detected is precisely an aesthetic feeling – the sublime that accompanies pleasure. What the critical philosopher fears above all is the somnolence of the thought process, the lack of 'play'. Pain and spasm, as is said in *The Conflict of the Faculties*, set the mind in motion, stimulate the activity of thought – the distraction of pain and insomnia. Kant, as an anthropologist, writes that 'pain is an incentive to activity'.[10] The pain of thinking pulls the philosopher out of his or her doctrinal somnolence, agitates the faculties and requires a judgement to settle conflict. Is life to recover its rights in this agitation? The generation by pain of the most general and diverse activities seems to be the opposite extreme of the conception developed by Christianity. Christianity urges us to the fundamental passivity of Christ enduring his exemplary suffering on the cross. This unique suffering – the Passion of Christ – redeems the human faults of mankind. Forgiveness and redemption are conceivable, worthy of hope and expectation as soon as the sense and the value of pain are ascribed to an end which exceeds the temporal life of man. But this passivity takes advantage of pain itself. The mediation of sin through pain implies the installation by pain of an activity that prayer and meditation display. It is in proportion to this meditation that Pascal suggests 'a good use of diseases' and recommends a 'good use' of the time of pain and individual suffering.[11] In this transaction – this exchange of pain and sin – there is a kind of obstinacy to find out a solution to the utmost suffering. But this obstinacy, or the pascalian recommendation as well, ignores what Emanuel Levinas calls the 'ultimate' of suffering – its exposure to the being, the ontological exposure to life and death simultaneously.[12]

What has just been mentioned about pain only refers to one's own suffering, to one's own pain. The threat of death, which pain welcomes, limits the promises of suffering, so to speak, to a relationship of the self to the self. But if the threat of death refers to the suffering of others, how is it possible to praise suffering and illness for the purpose, justified by authorities, of torture and other cruelties? After extermination or 'Gulag' camps, how are we to regard the suffering of peoples and individuals? And when death or the threat of death reaches a climax, i.e. theodicy or ideology, in the name of what is suffering endured or accepted? What is left of pain but its hateful uselessness?

1 Cf. Plato, *Pheidon*, 60 c.

2 Cf. Lucretius, *De la Nature* Livre 11 (*On Nature*, Book 11).

3 Cf. Epicurus, Sentences Vaticanes (*The Vatican Judgements*).

4 Cf. Bergson, *Matière et Mémoire* (*Matter and Memory*). PUF, 1959.

5 Cf. Kant, *Anthropology du Point de Vue Pragmatique* (*Anthropology from a Pragmatic Point of View*) p. 60. VRIN, 1970.

6 Cf. Hervé Guibert, *L'homme au Chapeau Rouge* (*The Man with the Red Hat*). Gallimard, 1992.

7 Cf. Plato, *The Republic*, L. VII.

8 Cf. Robert Jaulin for instance, in *La Mort, Sara* (Death, Sara); and Pierre Clastres, in *La Société contre l'Etat* (*Society against the State*).

9 Cf. Kant, *Essai pour Introduire en Philosophie le Concept de Grandeur Négative* (*An Essay in Order to Introduce the Concept of Negative Magnitude in Philosophy*). VRIN, 1949.

10 Cf. Kant, *Anthropology*, Ibid.

11 Cf. Pascal, *Prière pour Demander à Dieu le Bon Usage de Maladies* (*Prayer to Ask of God for the Good Use of Illnesses*), Pléiade, Editions Gallimard, 1954.

12 Cf. Emanuel Lévinas, *Le Temps et l'Autre* (*Time and the Other*). 'Quadrige', PUF, 1985; *Entre Nous* (*Between Us*). 'Figures'. Grasset, 1991.

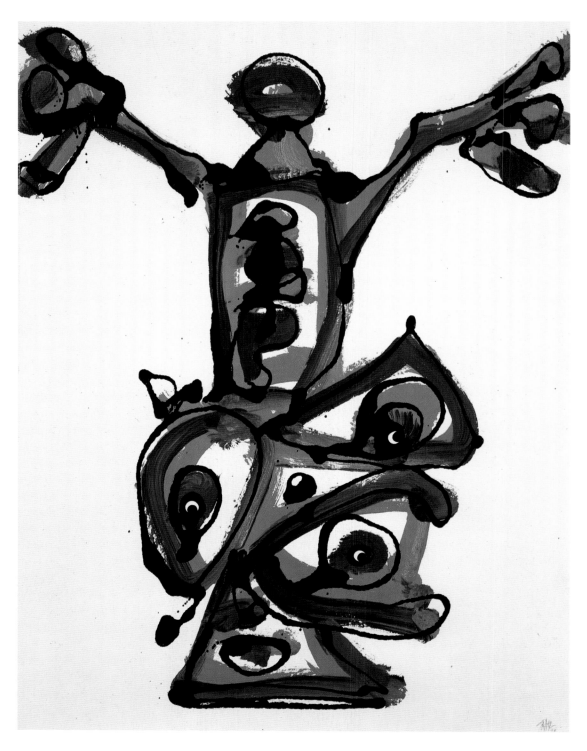

A. Saura.
Ecorché.
(Galerie Stadler)
(Ph. François Poivret)

Mad with Pain

Representations of pain in psychoanalysis

Patrick Lacoste

THE 'mad' we do not understand; those 'mad with pain' we understand too well. From one and the other, we discreetly withdraw, protecting ourselves in the guise of common sense. There are good reasons to claim that an acute and intractable pain can drive the most normal individual 'mad'. But what is the nature of the kind of pain that does not express the usual logic of the body, a pain that is intractable? Would the body's common sense misunderstand

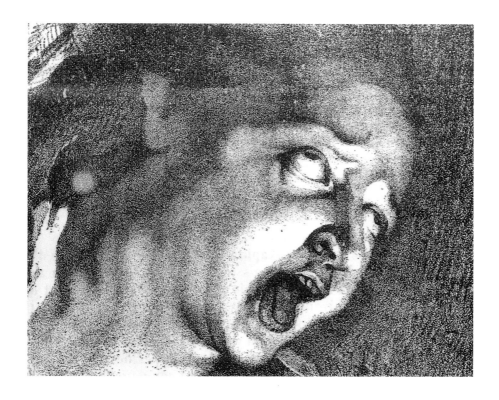

Study of a head. Facsimile of a lithography by J. Scarlett Davis, based on an original painting by Rubens. (M. Charcot Collection) (Centre de l'Image – AP-HP)

147

such 'dull' pain? The accepted model of physical sensation necessarily calls for a conscious realisation of pain. In addition to the psychological effect of the slightest physical pain, psychoanalysis distinguishes between psychogenic pain of the body, neurotic pain and psychotic pain. The sources or components of these types of pain are not conscious; they also entail unconscious pain.

The nerves have for a long time laid out a projection of the body in the use of language. The science of anatomy took a long time to show this projection in detail, which the science of neurology then found difficult to accommodate. This projection of the body acknowledges its psychical origins but often prefers to ignore them.

Many scientific discoveries have succeeded in representing pain and in reviving the secular debate on the relationship between the body and the spirit. They have, incidentally, also succeeded in always referring to the 'soul' for its less physical aspects. Being a materialism of the 'psychical device', which does not neglect hallucinations and fantasies and claims to be suspicious of conscience and perception, psychoanalysis can only disappoint those who fervently believe in objective description of painful mechanisms, especially since its 'instruments' of treatment (i.e. transfer and counter-transfer) are not painless. The greatest pain is the 'dull' kind, they say; but it can be painful sometimes simply to talk, especially when the memory expresses little and yet betrays quite a lot with regard to the perceptions and sensations of the spoken word.

What would be the exact assessment of the progress of anaesthesia nowadays, in comparison with that of torture and massacres? Who would dare denounce, beyond the considerable benefits of analgesics, the ideological drift transforming the useful prevention of pain into the marketing of useless precautions? Failing a therapeutic success, what lessons can be drawn from the position of the drug addict at the centre of the unlikely equation where more pleasure equals less pain? Finally, when the urgency of physical pain presses from all sides, when obtaining the best sensations is still the goal and when antidepressants – not to mention anxiolytics – are considered a panacea, what is the relationship we have with the slightest incentive to think about the psychical and its pain?

In a panorama of small pangs, it seems that human beings still prevail over the worst of their own creation. One would still have to fear that curiosity concerning psychical pain may be nothing else but a depressed or perverted version of the quest for pleasure. Thus, psychoanalysis, which tends to consider that a painful or depressive moment perhaps represents the only chance for an individual to take time out to think about him or herself, would not be regarded as a 'good' discourse when compared with the soothing discourses made in the name of progress.

The fact remains that this revival of interest in physical pain and the discoveries which followed it are essentially the result of research on objective and

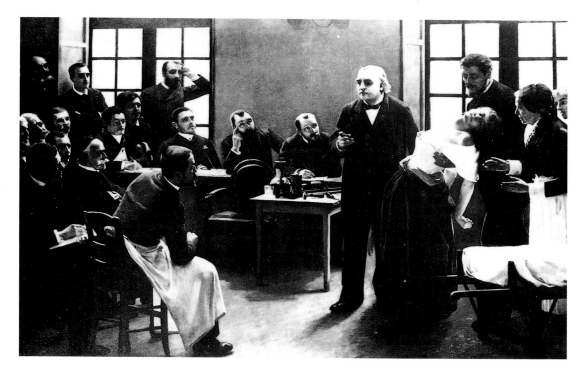

Lecture by Charcot.

harmful negative perceptions, and that this physiology of nociception is to the human problem of pain what the physiology of sexual activity is to pleasure, erotism, and perhaps to love; i.e., a necessary component of it, but only a component. As the proverb goes: 'I could not care less about what I do not know'. We all believe we have become experts regarding what is harmful to ourselves, even though we are all confronted with the same enigma and the same impossibility of finding out and understanding what makes us feel good. This is true in so far as we can objectively tell. Therefore, contrary to all expectations, psychoanalysis claims to uphold a materialism of that which is out of measure, which cannot be measured but in terms of a language itself boundless.

Representations of the Issue

What is pain for the psychical? And the pain is what is in question. The issue of pain would at once be party to an ignorance that escapes us. At the beginning of the research, we fail to agree on the formulation of the question because we believe that, through our own experience, we know the nature of pain. As a result, we long pay the price for this negligence by disagreeing among ourselves, because the disagreement is within us. We will actively be seeking to force into reason that which is beside reason. If we start from the known, and move into two directions, there are at least two logics. First, we begin with what is fairly well known to us and then we move on to what is very well known to us. It would be worth going over all of Western philosophy with regard to this particular theme. But one can postulate, except for a few variations, that the issue has remained 'Greek' in relative as well as in absolute terms. Only the martyr and the mystic would have tried to go against this line of thought and to substitute it with a body that is imagined in the name of incarnation.

Supposing that reminiscing can make one suffer, that the body of the hysterical, when stirred up by an inaccessible recollection, is legible as a special language – i.e. a physical pain for a psychical suffering, the first symbolic contract that Freud proposes for the symptom of hysteria is the following: the expression of the body would have drawn from the same sources as language. Hence, the expression 'a blow to the heart' can lead to cardiac pain, just like not being able to 'swallow' an affront may be translated into dysphagia.

By determining the effect of a psychical representation that could not be formulated in any other way but via the symptoms, and first through the body, Freud tried to turn the subjective into the objective, setting the intimate at the centre of a scientific psychology. This form of psychology would not confine itself – like that of Taine – to understanding the connection between a molecular movement and a sensation, but would aim at establishing the molecular status of a sensation for the thoughts, whether the conscience is present to perception or not. Familiar pains and strange thoughts thus combine in a kind of subjectivity that, for the analyst, is never obvious at the beginning. The contrast between the objective and the subjective is dependent upon a development whereby the part of acquisition of negation is anything but slight. This means that the very make-up of the psychical system cannot be achieved without pain either.

The apparent irreducibility between the physical and psychical inscriptions vanishes in the view that language may only be a consequence of the cry. Initially learnt from the attempt to master the external world for better protection against the inner world, it may be required by development as well as evolution. This was until Freud realised that the inner world knew how to take its revenge on the body, from the constraints of language and the mind which neglected it.

In order to bring together the aesthetic debates, with a view to understanding the aesthetic itself, one could say for instance that, if the work of Edvard Munch (*The Cry*) – almost contemporaneous with *Etudes sur l'Hystérie* (*Studies on Hysteria*) – seems to contradict the postulate of Lessing on the mystery of the cry, then the implementation of the functions of speech and language by Freud challenges the radical and almost automatic presupposition of what the expression of physical pain is (as a psychical model), while the sensation remains one of the possible alphabets of pleasure.

Neither the metaphor nor the lyricism would exempt us from recalling an adjacent examination of the openness of each language to the words at its disposal or those that it creates concerning pain. Moreover, the inner relation-

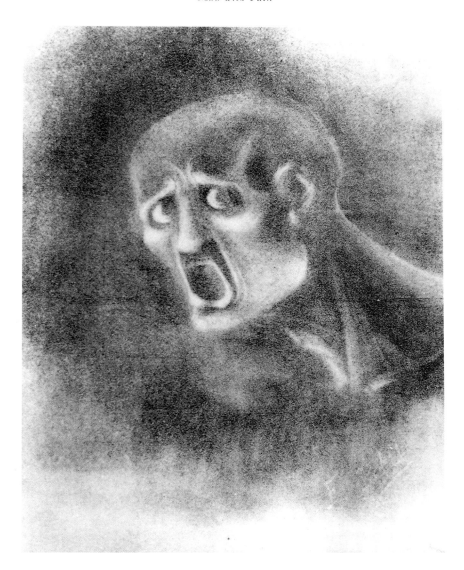

Hallucination of terror. Drawing made at
the beginning of dementia praecox.
(Collection of M. le D. Sicard)
(Centre de l'Image – AP- HP)

ships of a language facing another certainly follow paths of variable length that have nothing in common. Hence, the French words *dolour* and *deuil* share etymology and sound effects which are obviously not shared in English by the words *pain* and *mourn*, nor in German by *Schmerz* and *trauer*.

It should be noted, for the record, that, at the end of the nineteenth century, Littré was still complaining about the disappearance of the French verb se douloir (to mourn), conjugated at the time as *nous nous deuillons* (we are mourning), the reflexive form of which represented a perhaps excessive economy of meaning.

From Onomatopoeia to Moaning

The minimal expression of pain is both a stereotyped and discreetly rich one. Where the stereotype of an ouch! ensures the signal – even for the individual who would not miss the opportunity of the slightest chance to speak to himself or herself briefly – onomatopoeia can put emphasis on the small event, as if to show language its modest beginnings in the phonation, to call the body to order or indeed even to insult the will for having slackened its vigilance. These collusions of motivity, of the sensorial and practical intelligence and even of self-accusation, will possibly be followed by the 'bad mood' of a short depressive moment, unless a reflection on the failed experience emerges. Pain will at once speak a different language, a secret language that one anticipates more clearly in discovering, not without surprise, that the smallest words of sensation must also be submitted to the translation of the foreign language; as if the onomatopoeia of pain were presupposed to be part of a spontaneous Esperanto.

One would be tempted to read the hysterical conversion as an onomatopoeia of the anatomy of a body initially disoriented by erogenous excitement, if it were not for the fact that onomatopoeia can significantly overload any speech within the capabilities of the tremendous concessions that the repressed dissatisfaction requests from the body while entrusting it exclusively with its representation.

Psychoanalysis has also progressively brought to light the fact that the ability to think can be reached through a dialectical form of hysteria; for instance, through obsessions and constraints, where the words take shape in the thoughts, like foreign elements, for the flow of representations, and where psychical life becomes the scapegoat of thought and language in order to avoid the sudden appearance of emotions. 'There is nothing, including hate, that cannot take the shape of a word', writes Freud about the Rat Man. A function of speech and language that is naturally analgesic – the expressive reaction to a pain is first an attempt to find self-relief – has become more paradoxical as one proceeds with this realisation of the suffering, the torments of the obsessed. In the process, the linguistic instrument discovers its dark side as it faces psychical pain, by moaning, and so produces a lesser pain. The more this moaning distorts

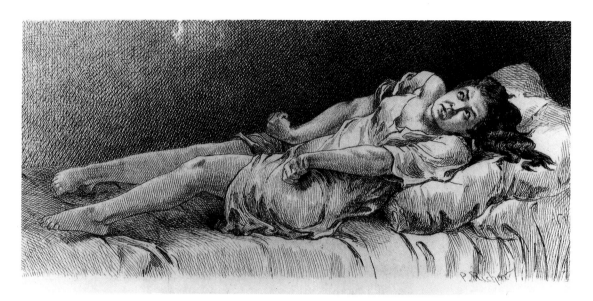

Phase of tonic immobility or tetanism.
(Centre de l'Image – AP-HP)

and represses the original pain the more the self becomes aware of this effect.

This perhaps tends to show that the psychical system, like the body, distinguishes between acute pain and chronic pain, but that its defences, because they are relational and linguistic, contrary to those of the body, can transform chronic pain into acute pain. Hence, psychotherapists acknowledge the intensity of the chronic.

The problems of psychosis, especially the function of delirium, is more obscure from this point of view. As a 'spontaneous attempt to heal', delirium can be a sign of psychical pain, but especially for the outsider, because it loses at once its function as a signal for those who suffer from it. It is remarkable that a number of accessible representations can be integrated, by way of diverting their meanings, into such a hermetic re-covering of psychical pain. This is because words can be dealt with as if they were things in these representations. For the schizophrenic for instance, the word 'hole' is a hole imprinted into the very texture of the psychical. For the paranoic it is also because words can represent the whole aggression of the world by projection, the object of love having become the persecutor. Thus, from a 'fundamental language' that would make public the 'murder of the soul', words can also suppress the body from these representations and quickly get caught in the shadow of the object on the self in the case of melancholics, whose speech seems forever veiled in mourning whereas their thoughts have never been clearer for their own misfortune.

This brief discussion can only outline, with psychoanalysis, the overall perspective of turning away from the mixed forms of neurosis – where the body remains audible even through a delayed expression – to the most acute forms of psychic pathology where the relationship with the body is either too distant or too close, because still in the service of a disguised rupture.

The Poles of Pain

The concept of 'somatic complacency' has been the subject of debate for a long time. The Freudian proposal that it concerns an encounter between the psychical and the body (and vice versa) has not made much headway. The conditions of this encounter are special every time it occurs. It is known that, on the one hand, the reduction of physical pain or psychical suffering does not necessarily mean the suppression of moaning. On the other hand, when increased by moaning, which in fact aims at reducing it, pain can become the organisational axis of the individual or of life. Therefore the poles of pain are at once joined together and divided according to the dead ends of pulsive and existential destinies.

Those who investigate hysteria constantly come up against the hypothesis and the role of an organic support for neurosis. Likewise, one would form the hypothesis of psychical supports in the old context of hypochondria or that of the numerous ailments which have since been brought under the blanket term of 'psychosomatic'. One must however distinguish, at the centre of the physical versus the psychological polemics concerning pain, the special and complex question posed by psychogenic pain.

Childhood provides knowledge about the physical force of 'scathing words', just as memory can differentiate gestures, slaps and small scratches according to the intensity of the psychological context generating recollection. It is not completely out of the question that the frequency of appendicectomies just before puberty may be considered as a new 'initiation rite' of civilised and sterilised societies. Physical pain is never the same through time, although its ability to surprise remains almost intact, as in the special case of the human being's relationship to the 'first time'. What would the algologist do with nostalgia? Psychogenic pain can draw from physical pain which makes up a biographical stock. Would there be, within the psychical, a mimesis of pain based on forgetfulness?

And yet, desire lives on the omission of its fulfilment in quest of the impossible accuracy of sensations of pleasure for the psychical. Excitement and tension are precisely bipolar models in the world of representations. The whole question of 'sexuality' in psychoanalysis is clearly focused on the closeness of the apparent relationship between learning about pain and the experience of pleasure. In the case of psychical pain, the experience would be as if radically cut off from any representation of possible alternation between tension and pleasure, or between pain and sedation.

Psychical pain comes under the sign of the irreparable and requires a complete reconstruction, not from the ruins, but next to or outside these ruins;

whereas psychogenic pain demands to be restored, and this demand is, in itself, the material needed for the restoration.

Physical Pains of Psychical Origin

Psychogenic pain takes up this territory at the frontier of physical and psychical pain. This frontier seems to have been extended as medicine was trying to define its own limits. In this area, Freud's theory only proposes the following precept:

'In the absence of any sign of reality, given that truth and fiction can equally carry some affects and, in some cases, be indistinguishable from one another, all that is left is to consider pain exclusively as the theme of a narrative, just like the dream, but without giving any preferential treatment neither to what would be attributable to physical adventure nor to what would present itself as a psychical event.'

Listening to pain as a narrative, but also listening to the associations that are the most devoid of sensorial tonality, as a possible path of painful awakening, is already a way of unveiling the function of delusion of the word for the memory and its ersatz function for sensation.

Psychogenic pain leads to the difficulty of evaluating the interference of the psychical on the different nerve impulses. It signals an intrapsychical conflict in which the representations of the body and the libidinous investment of these representations play an expressive role that the other modes are denied. It seems sensible to say that the psychical conflict is not the pain of the psychical but a tenacious protection against any risk of structural attack. It is in order to better hide the unspeakable weaknesses of the defences of the psychical or the poverty of the life of representations through this secret reinforcement, which becomes evident as a major inconvenience, that suffering recruits the body, at the price of some pain. Therefore, the conflict remains a support for the thought process against itself. And, paradoxically, the suffering that the conflict cannot restrain, takes shelter in a pain which is most often an elective one. Here, for want of explanations, the body serves as a means of interpreting the body itself.

The most frequently and easily located bases of the representations are generally the back and the anus for men and the stomach and the tongue for women. Dorsalgia and lumbago, anal pain, pelvic pain and 'essential glossodynia' would be the various degrees of a special scale of opacity, special in that the current great achievements of medical imagery find here an almost obstinate limit. The head, with the cephalea, in the case of both sexes, represents the summit of these psychogenic pains. A physical and/or psychological trauma is most often the starting point (to the point of sometimes being the only chance of autobiography). It is a trauma of (and for) the consciousness which is therefore only a form of pure luck for the determinism of a possible psychical trauma. Just as conspicuous, is the new trauma which is induced by painful weaning in cases where the body is allowed to respond to analgesics (without anyone being able to foresee their real effects).

The psychogenic path of pain implies a reallocation of the libido. The investment of sexual drive is withdrawn from the usual objects and from the external world, but the return to the self finds an ego that has been more or less altered. From the point of view of the withdrawal of the urge and its redistribution on the organ – as though narcissism had to be consolidated by a physical limit locking up the internal world – psychogenic pain would be the reverse of the psychological effect of physical pain. On the model quoted by Freud with regard to the poet's raging toothache, 'His soul is confined to a small hole on his molar', one could say that the representation of the molar is called for, summoned before the wide open chasm of the soul, in order, if not to fill it in, at least to draw its edges closer. The organ and the moan that gives it a name or underscores it both contain the external signifiers of this chasm which threatens the internal narcissism without having really reached it as yet.

There are cases of psychogenic pain resulting from a lack of preparation for mourning or a lack of further elaboration on the loss one has suffered. This can be a pathology of mourning which does not necessarily turn into a case of pathological mourning. Such pain, in spite of appearances, still spares the subject from meeting with what would be unbearable for the psychical.

Psychical Pain

What psychoanalysis tends to call 'psychical pain' is of a different nature than the psychological effect of physical pain and the double effect of psychogenic pain. Psychical pain would have to be examined from the point of view of a set of relational clues showing that narcissism has been affected. Neither the body nor language can really transmit this kind of pain. Psychical pain is the major sign of a significant, special and fundamental loss, of a loss which is neither an absence nor a disappearance. One would be tempted, beyond what the poetic lyricism or the tragic metaphor can offer, to be extremely restrained in this case. It is about approaching the nakedness of the being, beyond the spoken word and language, and it is so difficult to expose oneself to the encounter of something that no onomatopoeia, no embryonic narrative can translate, transpose or transmit from the rough state of silence, from a void in the ability of representation; it is a long silent cry as a form of presence by way of existence. To be just pain, faced with the impossibility of even having access to the 'pain of existing', goes beyond all the literature, because it goes beyond the very principle of pleasure.

Nevertheless, the great writers have sometimes brought us very close to this question of pain. Samuel Beckett is a case in point. He has turned into a new language the stripping of the misery of language itself. But, if Proust declares that 'suffering goes further in psychology than psychology itself' with

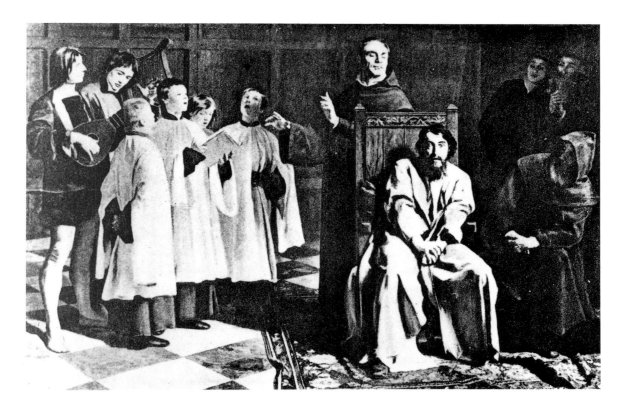

*E. Wauters. The Melancholy of the Painter
Hugo van der Goes (Brussels Museum).
(Centre de l'Image – AP-HP)*

regard to the disappearance of Albertine, his psychological perceptiveness concerning the disappearance of the object of love still does not tell us anything about a consciousness that no one would want; the strange consciousness resulting from a failure of the first model of the loss felt within the self – from the fact that the original relationship to the object that is always lost has not even been clearly and solidly established – for lack of sufficient constitution of this object for the psychical.

The disappearance, the absence, a common form of loss, presupposes the total existence of this 'lost object', the master of future investments in the object. When the first object – i.e. the mother, the 'first person', the closest human being – has constituted itself only as an object of need, and fails to allow for a transition from need to desire, self-esteem is definitely blocked. One can only lose what already existed and was represented as an object in the psychical, and all the more present in the psychical once it is lost; because the tragedy of the human psyche is that it is truly a founder, the loss of the first object being inescapable, only if the representations draw their intensity and vividness from this very loss.

That the lost object appears as 'a blank', that it has always been a shadow, that it is no more than a ghost in the constitutive archives of the internal world and the echo of a clearly intractable pain, echoes at once in the analytical course of treatment or increasingly shows through since there is a regression.

Now, the sketch of a violation of the elementary defences, now the primary masochism or the fact that it is not repressible in terms of the death instinct (thanatos), it offers itself to understanding and serves as the marker. Sometimes, the impossibility of giving up the pressure of the negative gives an orientation to the interpretation. But, always, this thing cannot be otherwise designated as a hole in the ability of being and of thinking which cannot be reduced to a blank in the memory. This 'hole' can always reveal itself, provided it can be identified, and confront the analyst with innate pain, with the brutal perspective of mourning that the mind must go through (or should have gone through) in order simply to start.

If Freud has constantly reminded us of this 'lost object', to be rediscovered and not to be found within reality, Lacan, on the other hand has discussed the notion of 'lack' at length, the notion of a rest (object a) as the components of the phases are being brought together. As a result, the psychoanalytic discourse is regularly exposed to misunderstanding, either by spreading (sometimes inordinately) the representations of an inherent 'negative', or by suggesting that normality, and even health, are reached when filling it.

Freud was always careful and reserved with regard to the approach of an interpretation of pain, although this was a persistent and often revived approach, and he even expressed doubts about this throughout his work. In this regard, perhaps we do not show quite as much surprise as we should concerning the inaugural confidences he made to Fliess on the fact that his intellectual work never 'succeeded' as much, except as a counterpoint of a physical malaise. So much so that a headache stimulated him and made him write. Perhaps we should also pay attention to the fact that, although suffering from cancer in the jaw since 1923, he did not stop publishing – and not works of lesser importance – when he was experiencing the most excruciating pain during the last sixteen years of his life.

In *Project for a Scientific Psychology* (1895), which he wrote while reading Taine and feeling very enthusiastic about the whole issue, Freud outlines a theory of physical pain as well as a theory of the psychical device. These outlines, which were not published in his lifetime, have been eleborated throughout the published works. First of all, Freud disputes the global model of the opposition between pleasure and pain put forth by contemporary and preceding psychologists. He proposes two alternative models. In one of these, the experience of satisfaction is governed by the principle of pleasure versus displeasure. In the other, pain is neither opposed to pleasure nor merged together with displeasure, but the experience of pain is quite simply defined in relation to the absence of pain which is obviously not assumed to be representable in the psychical, unless the zero of the 'return to zero' of tensions is given more weight than necessary.

Twenty years later, one can find confirmation of this notion of a difference between pain and displeasure in *Mourning and Melancholy* where the issue of a 'displeasure of pain' is discussed, because the expression confirms that the

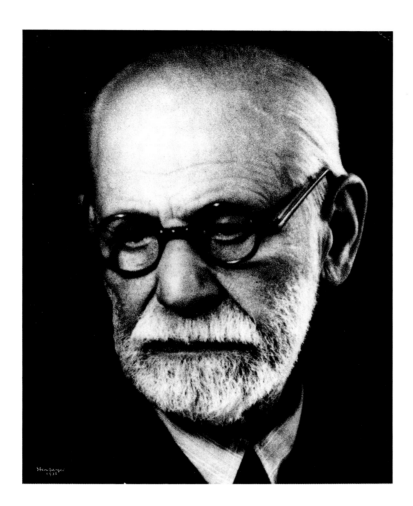

Sigmund Freud in 1938, at the age of 82.
(Mary Evans/Sigmund Freud Copyrights)

terms are not interchangeable – if not, why *describe* displeasure through pain?

The psychical experience of pain presupposes much more than the creation of tension. A boundary would have been crossed and a frontier would have been materially destroyed somewhere, by some quantity of energy. The limit of the self (as a physical and psychical self) is mainly at issue, because the regulation of the principle of pleasure and the principle of reality is just as fragile in the case of an external violation as it is in the case of an *internal* violation.

The external violation – and this is the problem with great traumas and the question of a compulsion of repetition and 'traumatophilia' – presents the additional risk of an internal release induced by it. The internal violation depends upon either a struggle between the authorities (i.e. the Ego, the Id and the Superego) – one authority can integrate the suffering of the other in terms of satisfaction – or of an inadequate differentiation between the authorities which, in turn, threatens individuals in their psychical structure. Furthermore, it is far from certain that, in cases where the limit does not really exist, the model of an internal violation would still be valid. The problem of masochism is of interest for both modes of violation, but the experience of pain is integrated in the principle of pleasure, until the internal or external accident occurs.

It has sometimes been pointed out that Freud's theorisation of the experience of pain referred back to the model of the affect (internal release). It is true that anxiety and guilt and love and hate can come with physical and psychogenic pain and lead to psychical pain. The pain of the psychical – just like pain in general can always lay, for the psychical, beyond the principle of pleasure – seems to be below the capacity of anxiety when the constitution of the psychical device remains within the subject. The experience of pain for the psychical can be compared to anguish, so long as there is a 'lost object', that object being, like the body, a peripheral source of pain for the self, but until a loss, in reactivating the lost object reveals a different type of loss, that is the narcissistic chasm in which it is the subject who gets lost.

What absolutely differentiates psychical pain from anguish in Freudian terms, is that the unconscious anguish will finally be reduced to the function of a mnemonic symbol – an archaic image that is supposed to be inscribed in the phylogenetic transmission – according to the conception of a universal capacity for anguish for the human being, while psychical pain is believed to isolate the individual who suffers from or bears it, both in the axis of development and in evolution.

If psychical suffering is half-way between anguish and mourning, then as a sign of the impossibility of reaching mourning, it is a testimony to the inconceivable mourning of the self as unaroused subject. In the first case, it is a question of avoidance. In the second, it is a question of cancellation. With some psychotics, there would be nothing psychical but for psychical cancellation. As well, the psychical is only concerned with the nullification of the body in some cases of melancholy. As long as psychical suffering still allows the body to become the psyche and, conversely, that the psyche can be perceived as the body (even though there is pain in the process) the edifice is under threat, more in terms of its balance than in terms of its very existence. Neurotic suffering uses conflicts and symptoms to avoid psychical pain which, from what has not been aroused, and with great persistence, nevertheless gives a sign of life, in spite of the cancellation or the vertigo of suppression.

Narcissism, while it can also be its agent or its producer, is always the last defence against psychical suffering. It remains the last frontier of the self for the mourning of the object, as well as for a serious attack on the body. Finally, narcissism is the container of the true distress signals, although it is eternally too exposed.

When an important psychical function is disabled, the suffering resulting from it does not allow for a distinction between the unconscious and the conscious, just as psychical pain reduces or suddenly causes any demarcation between the spirit and the body to disappear. Hence, the repression that was considered useful, and with good reason, gives way when faced with the pressure of the repressed or becomes even more pathogenic. Stratagems or blunders of repression cannot do much against psychical pain which does away with the precarious compartmentalisation or signals that it has not built. Since it lacks the capacity to expect any response from the object, even the lost object, the psychical thus accepts no further responsibility, starting with itself. If the real and reality, both internal and external, are not or are no longer usefully separated by the function and the distance of fantasy, the entire person does not exist any more, except as an admission of absence, taking the place of a 'presence of spirit'.

Psychical pain creates a presence made of absence without object which refutes the existence of the analyst in absorbing him or her in a catastrophe of transfer. As though drawn onto the site of a pain which ignores all substitutes, the analyst only has to be inspired by the suffering witnessed in others or recognised as his or her own, in order to try in spite of everything and, paradoxically, to create a conflict where there is none.

The representations of pain in psychoanalysis compel everyone to ask a number of questions. These questions would very much be like those of the architect (at the construction stage) if they were not too often raised after the event. In fact, the psychoanalytic treatment rebuilds the memory, but not without demolishing the clearest recollections. It reconstructs speech in language and the effect of representations, as well as the intensity of words on the body. This undertaking sometimes reaches down to the very foundations of the being, especially when it does not go straight to the point and does not target them intentionally.

For psychoanalysis, 'thinking' is a detour operation starting from the experienced dissatisfaction. Assuming that the psychical device is capable of hallucinating the satisfaction of the need, Freud has based the activity of thinking in displeasure and in the bringing into tension that it causes. But, if 'normal' hallucination seems to triumph for a while, the thoughts in effect represent no more than the progressive and substitute results of this primary recourse, a recourse that knows its limit in the duration of displeasure and acknowledges at once its weakness in the experience of pain. If the thought process *has* some constant recollections of dissatisfaction, it is in order to better forget its powerlessness in the face of the specific pain. It is the repository of psychical suffering, but only at the embryonic stage or continuously aborted in the face of psychical pain.

The psychical, unlike the body, does not know of any so-called exquisite pain which allows one to pinpoint the line of rupture with accuracy. Its lines of demarcation are nevertheless continuous, regardless of the outcome of its configuration. The ego is never in one block. The capacities of memory and speech, of love and thought, contain every day the fragility of these lines of demarcation that suffering and pain not only erode but can also induce (cleft lives).

In the face of what remains walled up in pain, psychoanalysis gives the illusion of reinforcing the wall of language, in order better to circumvent, use or go beyond it. Words for pain, regardless of their effects and origin, are really 'passwords' in the sense that they appease, at least for a while, the radical hate for the similar or self-hate. Those who have the word triumph over death in passing. It is the least that the human being can hope for and eventually gain from the living sciences and the social sciences. As for psychoanalysis, which is at the same time knowledge of man and of the living, its representations of pain commit the interprepation to continuously strive up to the level of the soaring moan.

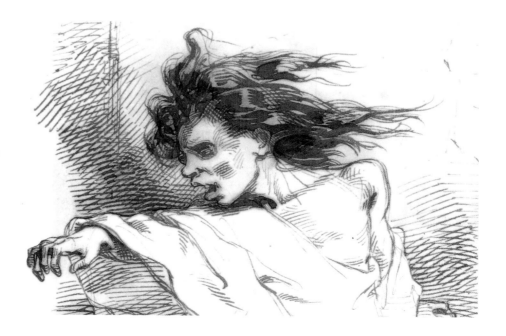

Chevalier Gavarni *(1804–1866).*
Insane. Pen and ink drawing.
(Centre de l'Image – AP-HP)

Bibliography

Neurobiology and Pain

Apicella, Paul *Guide illustré du neurone* Belin 1988

Canguilhem, G. *La santé: concept vulgaire* Sable 1990

Changeux, Jean-Pierre *L'homme neuronal* Fayard 1983

Catalogue of the exhibition 'L'homme transparent' Palais de la Découverte

Catalogue of the exhibition 'La fabrique de la pensée' Cité des Sciences et de L'Industrie

Melzack Ronald and Wall, Patrick D. *Le défi de la douleur* Edisem-Vigot 1989

Ninio, Jacques *L'empreinte des sens* Odile Jacob 1989

Peschanski, Marc *Biologie de la douleur* Collection *Science et Découvertes* le Rocher 1986

Snyder, Solomon *Drugs and the Brain* Pour la Science Belin 1987

The Brain Pour la Science 1981

Vincent, Jean-Didier *Biologie des passions* Odile Jacob 1986

Behaviour and Pain

Anzieu, Didier *Le Moi-peau* Dunod 1985

Bettelheim, Bruno *Psychanalyse des contes de fées (Psychoanalysis of Fairy Tales)* Robert Laffont 1976

Chanteur, Janine *Les petits-enfants de Job* Le Seuil 1990

Chapoutier, G. *Au bon vouloir de l'homme, l'animal* Denoël

Cyrulnik, Boris *Mémoire de singe et paroles d'homme* Hachette Pluriel 1984

Cyrulnik, Boris *Sous le signe du lien* Hachette 1989

Gauvain-Piquard, Annie *La douleur chez l'enfant* Medsi McGraw-Hill 1989

Meyers, Claude *Brève histoire des drogues et médicaments de l'esprit* Erès 1985

Montagner, Hubert *L'attachement, les débuts de la tendresse* Odile Jacob 1988

Pontalis, J.B. *Entre le rêve et la douleur* Gallimard 1977

Szasz, Thomas S. *Pain and Pleasure* Payot 1986

Widlöcher, Daniel *Les logiques de la dépression* Fayard 1983

Medicine and Pain

Boureau, François and Willer, Jean-Claude *La douleur, exploration, traitement par neurostimulation et électro-acupuncture* Masson 1982

Boureau, François *Contrôler votre douleur* Payot 1986

Debache, C. and Depoix R. *Accoucher sous péridurale* Collection Connaissance et Santé, Denoël 1989

Nguyen Van Nhan *Traitement de la douleur, acupuncture chinoise, électropuncture, digito-puncture* Simep 1989

Revault d'Allonnes, Claude *Le mal joli* Plon 1991

Saunders, Dame Cicely and Baines, Mary *Life helping death* Medsi 1986

Soum, Pierre *La douleur est inutile* Favre 1982

Traitement de la douleur cancéreuse OMS 1987

Pharmacology and Pain

Couturier, M. *La douleur, place des antalgiques* Editions de L'Interligne 1990

Eschwège, E., Bouvenot G., Doyon F., Lecroux A. *Essais thérapeutiques, mode d'emploi* Inserm 1990

Lachaux, B. and Lemoine P. *Placebo, un médicament qui cherche la vérité* Medsi McGraw-Hill 1988

Pignarre, Philippe *Ces drôles de médicaments* Collection Les empêcheurs de tourner en rond, Laboratoires Delagrange 1990

Solignac, Pierre *Merveilleuse asprine* M.A. Editions

Directives pour le contrôle des stupéfiants et des substances psychotropes OMS 1986

Développement et évaluation du médicament Third Inserm Symposium-DPhM, PLM 26 – 29 January 1987

Anthropology and Pain

Hainard J. and Kaehr R. (editors) *Le mal et la douleur* Ethnography Museum of Neuchâtel 1986

Hirsch, Emmanuel *Médecine et éthique, le devoir d'humanité* Editions du Cerf, 1990

Literature and Pain

Brenot, Philippe *Les mots de la douleur* Bordeaux Le Bouscat, L'Esprit du Temps 1990

Le Clézio, J.M.G., *Le jour où Beaumont fit connaissance avec sa douleur* Mercure de France 1964

Duras, Marguerite *La douleur* P.O.L. 1985

Eluard, Paul *Capitale de la douleur* Gallimard

Rilke, Rainer Maria *Le livre de la pauvreté et de la mort* Actes Sud.

Vincent, J.D. *Casanova, la contagion du plaisir* Odile Jacob 1990